W9-DHM-205

Understanding Controversial Therapies
for Children with Autism,
Attention Deficit Disorder,
and Other Learning Disabilities

JKP Essentials

Understanding Motor Skills in Children with Dyspraxia, ADHD, Autism, and Other Learning Disabilities
A Guide to Improving Coordination
Lisa A. Kurtz
ISBN 978 1 84310 865 8

Visual Perception Problems in Children with AD/HD, Autism, and Other Learning Disabilities
A Guide for Parents and Professionals
Lisa A. Kurtz
ISBN 978 1 84310 826 9

Dyslexia and Alternative Therapies
Maria Chivers
ISBN 978 1 84310 378 3

Understanding Regulation Disorders of Sensory Processing in Children
Management Strategies for Parents and Professionals
Pratibha Reebye and Aileen Stalker
ISBN 978 1 84310 521 3

Understanding Nonverbal Learning Disabilities
Maggie Mamen
ISBN 978 1 84310 593 0

Understanding Controversial Therapies for Children with Autism, Attention Deficit Disorder, and Other Learning Disabilities

A Guide to Complementary and Alternative Medicine

Lisa A. Kurtz

Jessica Kingsley Publishers
London and Philadelphia

First published in 2008
by Jessica Kingsley Publishers
116 Pentonville Road
London N1 9JB, UK
and
400 Market Street, Suite 400
Philadelphia, PA 19106, USA

www.jkp.com

Library of congress cataloging in Publication Data
Kurtz, Lisa A.
Understanding controversial therapies for children with autism, attention deficit disorder, and
other learning disabilities : a guide to complementary and alternative medicine / Lisa A. Kurtz.
   p. cm. -- (JKP essentials series)
   ISBN 978-1-84310-864-1 (pb : alk. paper) 1. Learning disabilities--Alternative treatment. 2.
Autism in children--Alternative treatment. 3. Attention-deficit hyperactivity
disorder--Alternative treatment. I. Title.
RJ496.L4K87 2008
618.92'85889--dc22

2007035919

British Library cataloguing in Publication Data
A CIP catalogue record for this book is available from the British Library

ISBN 978 1 84310 864 1

Printed and bound in the United States by
Thomson-Shore, Inc.

CONTENTS

Part 3. Resources for Children with Autism,
Attention Deficit Disorders, and Other
Learning Disabilities

PART 1

INTRODUCTION

Chapter 1

INTRODUCTION

Children with disabilities are at risk for experiencing problems in many aspects of their lives, including becoming independent in daily living skills, meeting academic expectations, learning to communicate, maintaining emotional and behavioral regulation, adapting to the social demands of society, and developing motor proficiency. Among children with disabilities, those with autism spectrum disorders, attention deficit disorders (ADD), and specific learning disabilities have received particular attention in the literature, and pose significant challenges to parents, teachers, and other professionals who hope to provide them with interventions that best ameliorate their difficulties.

Professionals who diagnose these disorders understand that certain defining traits or characteristics are used to determine if a child "fits" the criteria for a particular diagnosis, and have developed protocols for testing and clinical assessment that can strongly suggest or confirm a diagnosis. For example, all children with autism spectrum disorders demonstrate problems impacting social reciprocity, communication, and behavior. Children with ADD display developmentally inappropriate levels of inattention or hyperactivity that are not related to medical or social-emotional factors, and that cause impaired adaptive performance at home, in school, or in situations requiring social interaction. Children with specific learning disabilities demonstrate a significant discrepancy between their ability to learn (based upon measures of intelligence) and their actual learning, and this discrepancy cannot be attributed to medical, economic, cultural, or social disadvantages that might account for the discrepancy. However, within each of these diagnostic groups, an enormous number of individual differences exist. Some children with autism learn to talk, while others must be trained to use non-verbal forms of communication. Many children with ADD are hyperactive, but others have under-responsive attention systems, and are lethargic and slow to respond to learning challenges. Children with specific learning disabilities exhibit wide variability as to their cognitive strengths and weaknesses, learning styles, and response to various curricula and instructional methods. Some children struggle with motor coordination or speech articulation, while others do not. Furthermore, some children with developmental disabilities may have related or concomitant disorders that complicate their individual profile. The presence of hearing or vision impairments, emotional disturbances, or other medical conditions greatly influences the impact of the disability on the child's ability to cope and to learn. Finally, factors such as the child's personality and temperament, emotional resilience, the strength and commitment of family support, and the availability and affordability of appropriate services can also greatly influence the unique prognosis for each individual child.

With such wide variety in the learning styles and differences among these children, it is no surprise that professionals have yet to agree upon the best practices for intervention. Certainly, guidelines do exist. There is significant pressure within medical and educational communities to provide treatment that is based upon scientific evidence of success and that focuses on relevant outcomes (sometimes called *evidence-based practice*). This typically requires that the specific intervention is isolated from other interventions, and is then subjected to a controlled study in which researchers look at the outcome of children who are randomly selected to receive the targeted intervention as compared with children who receive an alternative or no intervention. Because the researchers are not told which children are receiving the targeted intervention, this is known as a *blind study*. Treatments that have been subjected to multiple blind studies that successfully document effectiveness, and that are then put through rigorous review and critique by professional peers so that the results can be published in reputable journals are often then accepted into conventional or mainstream medical or educational practices. However, many types of intervention for children with developmental disabilities do not lend themselves easily to this type of study. Because of the variability of individual characteristics in children with disabilities, it is often hard to put together a group of children who are similar enough to be considered a "unique" group. If there is too much variability in the study group, and some subjects improve while others do not, it is hard to know whether the changes that are observed relate to the intervention or to individual differences among members of the study group. Also, many studies take place over a period of weeks, months, or longer. If improvement occurs, it is difficult to demonstrate whether improvement is attributable to normal maturation as opposed to the effects of the intervention. Furthermore, many interventions for developmental disabilities are dynamic in nature, requiring the development of a therapeutic rapport with the child, along with active participation on the part of the child, family, and others involved with the child. These personal variables are difficult to control in a scientific study. This makes scientific study of developmental interventions potentially more complicated than the study of effectiveness of a specific drug, exercise, surgery, or other more concrete type of intervention.

The interventions that are commonly recommended by professionals may be governed by a variety of regulatory practices that have been developed in consideration of scientific evidence. In the United States, federal and state regulations offer standards and guidelines for providing services within early intervention and educational settings (see Individuals with Disabilities Education Improvement Act (IDEIA) 2004). In the United Kingdom, a government code of practice, the Special Educational Needs and Disability Act 2001, offers guidance to local education authorities and state schools on how to identify, assess, and monitor students with special learning needs. Professionals who are licensed or otherwise regulated in their practice must operate within the scope of practice as defined by their profession or by local regulatory agencies. Also, the specific interventions recommended by professionals may or may not be covered under various insurance or other reimbursement agencies. All of these regulatory practices are designed to help to assure that children have access to treatments that meet approved standards of care and are likely to be effective.

This book is intended to offer parents and professionals a brief overview of certain non-conventional, controversial interventions that may be considered for children with developmental disabilities including autism spectrum disorders, attention deficit disorders, and specific learning disabilities. Its purpose is to help readers to understand the basic theory behind each intervention, the typical procedures involved, and where to go for more information about the intervention or about the qualifications of professionals using the intervention. It is in no way meant to endorse or condemn any of the interventions described, nor to offer medical or educational advice, but simply to help readers to expand their knowledge of available interventions. The interventions discussed offer a representative, but not comprehensive, overview of available therapies at the time this book was written. Resources listed in the appendix can offer readers a mechanism for staying informed about controversial therapies as scientific evidence is gathered about those interventions included in this book, or as other interventions become available.

REFERENCES

US Department of Education (2004) *Individuals with Disabilities Education Act (IDEIA)*. Available at http://thomas.loc.gov/cgi-bin/query/z?c108:h.1350.enr:, accessed on 3 December 2007.

Special Educational Needs and Disability Act (2001) London: The Stationery Office. Available at www.england-legislation.hmso.gov/acts.acts2001/ukpga_20010010_en_1, accessed 17 December 2007.

DISCLAIMER

This book is intended for informational purposes only, and is not meant to provide specific medical or psychoeducational advice. Opinions expressed are those of the author, and should not be taken as an endorsement nor condemnation of any intervention method or procedure. All decisions about treatment for children with disabilities should be made in consideration of the available scientific evidence for effectiveness and safety, and should be discussed with the child's pediatrician and other qualified professionals involved in the child's care. The author disclaims all liability, loss, injury, or damage incurred directly or indirectly as a result of use of any information contained in this book.

Chapter 2

THINKING OUT OF THE BOX

*An Overview of Complementary
and Alternative Medicine Approaches*

Medicine can be described as the practice of maintaining or restoring health through the study, diagnosis, and treatment of disease and injury. *Conventional medicine* refers to the provision of medical care as shared by *doctors* (Medical Doctors or MDs, and Doctors of Osteopathy or DOs) and by *allied health professionals*, including nurses, psychologists, occupational therapists, speech-language therapists, physical therapists, and others. The practice of conventional medical care is regulated through various professional licensing and credentialing boards that assure the public of the competency of members. In conventional medicine, practices and interventions are based upon sound scientific research that proves both the efficacy and safety of the intervention. These interventions are therefore widely accepted among the broad medical community. Conventional medicine may also be referred to as *Western medicine, orthodox medicine, mainstream medicine* or *allopathy*.

Complementary and Alternative Medicine (CAM) refers to a diverse array of health care systems, practices, and interventions that are not considered to be part of conventional medicine. Although interventions included in this category may have undergone research and may have popular acceptance among consumers, there are generally insufficient data available to assure the outcome and safety of the interventions. Training in the use of CAMs can be highly variable, in some cases leading to credentialing, such as licensure for massage therapists, or voluntary certification in certain auditory training programs. Unfortunately, however, it is not uncommon for professionals to incorporate use of CAMs as part of their practice with little or no formal training. In fact, some lay personnel practice interventions with virtually no formal professional training or credentialing, and with a very limited under-standing of the basic concepts underlying the health and psychosocial well-being of their clients. The list of interventions that are considered to be CAMs undergoes continual change as some are proven effective and are adopted by conventional medical practice, while newer therapies and interventions are proposed and introduced to the public.

Although complementary and alternative medical practices are often referred to together as CAMs, there are important distinctions between the two. *Complementary medicine* refers to interventions that are used along with more con-ventional treatment. For example, yoga might be used to achieve a calm and relaxed state prior to a challenging physical therapy exercise program, or aromatherapy might be used to promote alertness prior to a reading instruction session for a child with learning disabilities. The practice of using safe combina-tions of conventional and non-conventional medicine is sometimes referred to as *integrative medicine. Alternative medicine* is used to describe interventions that take the place of traditional medicine, for example, seeking treatment from a homeo-pathic physician instead of an MD or DO, or using elimination diets as a substi-tute for prescription medication to reduce hyperactivity in children with attention deficit disorder. The use of CAMs has gained increasing popularity in recent years, especially as there is greatly increased access to information about therapeutic options through the Internet. For parents of children with lifelong developmental differences, frustration with slow progress using more tradi-tional approaches, or limited access to those services, may encourage them to seek other answers. Parents may also choose to explore the use of CAMs based upon the recommendations of friends or professionals they trust, or based upon personal beliefs and traditions. For example, less invasive therapies may be attractive to parents who fear the potential side effects of drugs used in conven-tional medicine, or they may find it easier to support a therapeutic intervention that is consistent with their own activity preferences, such as music, dance or martial arts. In fact, according to the National Institutes of Health, more than one-third of adults in the United States use some form of complementary or alternative medicine (Barnes *et al.* 2004). Most doctors of conventional medicine are open to discussing the use of CAMs with patients and their families, and some will consider making a referral under the right circumstances. Other physicians, however, are cautious about recommending alternative treatments due to their susceptibility for medical liability (American Academy of Pediatrics 2002).

In 1992, the United States Congress created the National Center for Com-plementary and Alternative Medicine (NCCAM) as one component of the

National Institutes of Health. This organization classifies CAM therapies into five categories or domains. The subsequent chapter presents a description of selected CAMs organized according to this model. The five domains are described as follows:

1. *Alternative Medical Systems*, based upon complete systems of theory and practice, such as homeopathic medicine or Ayurveda.

2. *Mind-body Interventions.* These use a variety of techniques designed to enhance the mind's capacity to affect bodily functions and symptoms (for example, meditation or creative arts therapies).

3. *Biologically-based Therapies*, which use substances found in nature, such as herbs, foods, and vitamins.

4. *Manipulative and Body-based Methods*, which are based on manipulation and/or movement of one or more parts of the body, such as chiropractic or massage.

5. *Energy Therapies*, involving the use of energy fields. There are two types of energy fields, *Putative (*also called *Biofields),* which purportedly surround and penetrate the human body but cannot be measured, and *Veritable*, which involve measurable wavelengths and frequencies of sound, light, magnetism, or other types of rays from the electromagnetic spectrum.

Parents and professionals who consider the use of CAMs for children with autism, attention deficit disorder, learning disabilities, or other disabilities or health care concerns should use caution when making such an important decision. Some CAMs have undergone at least some promising research to demonstrate effectiveness, but all CAMs included in this book should be considered unproven, at least as of the writing of this book. It is easy for parents and professionals alike to be fooled into thinking a treatment "works" when there are many anecdotal claims of success and media attention. However, *placebo effect* may, in fact, be behind many claims of success. Placebo effect refers to the perception of positive outcomes of an intervention that may or may not be due to the actual intervention. This can occur because with any intervention, scientifically proven or not, positive things usually happen. The professional enters into a relationship with the child and family and gets to know them on a personal level. He or she can then answer questions, offer helpful guidance about daily issues or problems, and provide emotional support and optimism. All of this is good, and can actually help the child to improve, but it may have nothing to do with the actual intervention, per se. This is not to say that placebo effect is necessarily bad, just that it warrants thoughtful consideration. Sometimes, children who undergo a new treatment make gains simply because they feel "special" or singled out, causing them to be more motivated and to work harder at improving their skills. In general, it would seem wise to first try scientifically validated, conventional interventions before considering the use of CAMs.

When CAMs are considered, the following guidelines are suggested for professionals:

- Search carefully for evidence as to the potential effectiveness and safety of the intervention before incorporating a CAM into your practice. It is your responsibility to know what evidence exists, and to judge the quality of that evidence. Anecdotal reports of effectiveness are not sufficient for making treatment decisions.

- Consider whether the CAM fits within the scope of practice as defined by your profession and by regulatory agencies. It is your ethical responsibility to practice within defined guidelines if you represent yourself as offering a professional service and expect to seek reimbursement as such.

- If you are employed by an agency (e.g. hospital, school system, rehabilitation center), know the agency's policy on CAMs before recommending an intervention.

- Never imply to a parent that they must agree to your recommendation. Your professional responsibility is to inform parents of the range of options available to them, and to discuss the pros and cons of the various options to the best of your ability.

- Obtain information from insurance agencies or other payors to determine coverage prior to recommending a CAM. The potential cost of an intervention should be an important factor for parents who must make difficult decisions about their child's care.

- Assure competency by obtaining the appropriate training/education before attempting to use the CAM. Some interventions require specific licensure or credentialing, while others do not. You are responsible for understanding standards of care expected for the intervention and striving to meet those standards. Never falsely represent yourself as an expert.

- Always consult with the child's pediatrician and other specialists for information on the CAM in question. Best practice dictates the importance of working as a team when making treatment decisions.

Also, it is extremely important to consider any potential for side effects or complications of the intervention based on the child's unique profile and other treatments that the child receives.

- Clearly communicate all risks and benefits associated with the proposed CAM to parents and, if appropriate, to the child. Besides potential health complications, use of unproven treatments may require the child and family to expend time and energy that could be more usefully applied towards other efforts.

- Be clear to parents in describing the anticipated outcomes of the intervention, and discontinue the intervention as soon as it appears to be ineffective. If the intervention appears to be helping, consider safely withdrawing the intervention for a period of time to see if there is decline, then re-establishing the intervention to be sure that it is, in fact, contributing to the observed changes.

Some considerations for parents who are investigating controversial therapies:

- Never expose yourself to the disappointment of seeking a "cure" for a developmental disability. If there was a treatment that could create miraculous changes in your child, your primary doctor would know about it. This does not mean that you should not consider controversial approaches to help your child achieve a better quality of life—just remind yourself to have reasonable expectations.

- Be an informed consumer. It is easy to become excited about a new intervention that shows promise based upon a friend's personal recommendation, a TV show, or a popular parent magazine. Research the intervention to your fullest ability, and discuss it with all of the trusted professionals you know. Look for arguments on both sides of the question, and carefully consider the opinions of those opposed to the intervention as well as those who support it. Internet resources that end with .edu or .gov often present more objective and scientifically valid descriptions of an intervention than those ending with .org or .com. If professionals are not in support of the intervention you are interested in, ask them for their specific reasons why. If you are not satisfied with their answers, consider asking for a second opinion.

- Remember that more therapy is not necessarily better therapy. For every intervention you pursue, there are multiple costs. Besides the potential for significant out-of-pocket expenses, the time and energy spent in pursuing the intervention, and the mental effort expended in anticipating improvement, can take a toll on parents and other family members.

- Be sure that you know what the cost will be before undertaking any new therapy. Often parents are understandably eager to start a new intervention, and are willing to pay in advance until their insurance is billed. Remember, however, that many CAMs are not covered by insurance, and insurance companies can be slow to make decisions regarding coverage. Some parents spend large amounts of money only to find that their insurance company has rejected the claim months after therapy was initiated.

- Ask the professional what his or her training and experience is in use of the CAM. Be wary of professionals who tell you that they learned the technique through inservice training or mentorship with peers when formal training or certification programs exist. Ask what successes they have seen with use of the intervention, and consider asking whether the professional can put you in touch with other families they have serviced.

- Ask the professional exactly what will occur during the course of the intervention so that you feel completely comfortable with the procedures that will take place and can explain them to your child. Ask what role you will be expected to take. Some interventions require you to purchase special tools or materials which can be costly. Some will require you to spend large amounts of time carrying over therapy techniques at home. Do not begin an intervention that you are unable to fully support.

- Ask the professional to explain how you will know that the intervention is working. Look for specific, measurable goals, and a timeline for achieving those goals. Ask frequently for the professional's opinion as to the effectiveness of the intervention, and do not be embarrassed to discontinue any intervention you feel is not working.

- Remember to take the time to enjoy your child for all the special qualities he or she has to offer, despite the disability. Parents who spend excessive time searching for a cure can lose sight of the unique pleasures involved in raising a child with special needs.

REFERENCES

American Academy of Pediatrics (2002) *Periodic Survey #49: Complementary and Alternative Medicine (CAM) Therapies in Pediatric Practices.* Available at www.aap.org/research/periodic survey/ps49bexs.htm, accessed on 8 April 2006.

American Occupational Therapy Association (2005) 'Complementary and alternative medicine (CAM) position paper.' *American Journal of Occupational Therapy, 59,* 6, 653–655.

Barnes, P., Powell-Griner, E., McFann, K. and Nahin, R. (2004) CDC Advance Data Report #343. *Complementary and Alternative Medicine Use Among Adults: United States, 2002.* Available at www.medicinenet.com, accessed on 8 April 2006.

National Center for Complementary and Alternative Medicine *What is Complementary and Alternative Medicine (CAM)?* Available at http://nccam.nih.gov, accessed on 6 July 2007.

Practice Committee of the Section on Pediatrics, American Physical Therapy Association (2004) *APTA Section on Pediatrics Fact Sheet: Considering Interventions from Alternative & Complementary Medicine.* Available at www.pediatricapta.org, accessed 8 April 2006.

Schechtman, M. (2005) 'Controversial therapies in the treatment of young children with developmental disabilities: Medical perspective.' *Early Intervention Training Institute Newsletter, Rose F. Kennedy Center*, Winter 2005–2006, 1–3.

PART 2

SELECTED INTERVENTIONS

Chapter 3

ALTERNATIVE MEDICAL SYSTEMS

ACUPUNCTURE/ACUPRESSURE

Acupuncture is the practice of using very fine, sterilized (or disposable), stainless steel needles to stimulate certain areas in or near the skin. The needles are typically twirled, pulled in and out, or are electrically stimulated, and are then left in the skin for approximately 20 minutes. Sometimes, the insertion of needles is combined with the use of heat and herbs. *Acupressure* is a similar intervention, but uses hand and fingertip pressure instead of needles to produce the stimulation. *Shiatsu* is a specific type of acupressure that combines pressure points with massage techniques. In the Western world, these interventions are most commonly used to relieve pain and decrease stress, although some practitioners use a specialized form of acupuncture to the ear to produce improvements in children with learning disabilities and Attention Deficit Hyperactivity Disorder (ADHD). The origins of these practices are based upon ancient Chinese medical beliefs which differ greatly from modern scientific theories about health. In ancient China, there was no knowledge of anatomy and physiology, biochemistry, nutrition, or the mechanisms of healing. Diseases were not studied and classified. Instead, a person with illness was believed to lack balance with nature and its two opposing forces, *yin* and *yang*. Yin represents the passive feminine qualities of nature, and yang represents the aggressive masculine qualities. A diagnosis was based upon checking various pulses and examining the tongue. Interventions were selected on a trial and error basis, and were directed at re-establishing balance and harmony as symptoms resolved. Acupuncturists believe that there are 14 *meridians* that channel the flow of *life force*, also called *Ch'i* or *Qi*. The insertion of needles at designated points along these meridians, or pressure over the points, is believed to increase or decrease the flow of Ch'i.

Acupuncture and acupressure are not painful if administered correctly, although they may produce numbness and a tingling sensation. Some patients report feeling calmer or more energized after therapy. Because the needles used in acupuncture are sterilized and only minimally invade the skin, there is generally little risk of complication, although occasional serious side effects have been reported. Most often, treatment involves 10 to 12 sessions, with periodic follow-up to assure that balance has been maintained.

Training in acupuncture

Acupuncture/acupressure is not part of the traditional curriculum taught in American and European medical schools. However, some accredited medical schools do sponsor courses for physicians. Acupuncture is permitted in all states in the United States, although some states only permit licensed physicians to perform the treatments, while others allow lay practitioners (usually referred to as Certified Acupuncturists or Master Acupuncturists) to provide treatment with or without medical supervision. Some private insurance companies cover acupuncture if it is provided by a licensed physician.

The United Kingdom Department of Health is in the process of defining statutory regulation for acupuncturists.

Recommended resources for acupuncture/acupressure

Literature

Breuner, C.C. (2002) 'Complementary medicine in pediatrics: A review of acupuncture, homeopathy, massage, and chiropractic therapies.' *Current Problems in Pediatric and Adolescent Health Care*, *32*, 10, 353–384.

British Medical Association (2000) *Acupuncture*. London: Taylor & Francis.

Ding, L. (1992) *Acupuncture, Meridian Theory, and Acupuncture Points*. Berkeley, CA: Pacific View Press.

Lee, B.Y., LaRiccia, P.J. and Newberg, A.G. (2004) 'Acupuncture in theory and practice.' *Hospital Physician*, *40*, 11–18.

Lytle, C.D. (1993) *An Overview of Acupuncture*. Rockville, MD: US Food and Drug Administration, Center for Devices and Radiological Health.

Agencies, organizations, and websites

Accreditation Commission for Acupuncture and Oriental Medicine (ACAOM)
Maryland Trade Center #3, 7501 Greenway Center Drive, Suite 760
Greenbelt, MD 20770, USA
Telephone: +1 (301) 313-0855
Website: www.acaom.org

This is the national accrediting agency in the United States recognized by the United States Department of Education to accredit Master's level degree programs in acupuncture.

British Acupuncture Council
63 Jeddo Road
London W12 9HQ, UK
Telephone: +44 (0)20 8735 0400
Website: www.acupuncture.org.uk
This is the main regulatory body for acupuncturists in the United Kingdom.

British Medical Acupuncture Society
12 Marbury House
Higher Whitley, Warrington, Cheshire WA4 4JA, UK
Telephone: +44 (0)1925 730727
Website: www.medical-acupuncture.co.uk

National Certification Commission for Acupuncture and Oriental Medicine (NCCAOM)
11 Canal Center Plaza, Suite 300
Alexandria, VA 22314, USA
Telephone: +1 (703) 548-9004
Website: www.nccaom.org
This organization offers a certification process for acupuncturists in the United States.

The British Medical Acupuncture Society
BMAS House, 3 Winnington Court
Northwich, Cheshire CW8 1AQ, UK
Telephone: +44 (0)1606 786782
Website: www.medical-acupuncture.co.uk
This is an association of medical practitioners promoting the use and scientific understanding of acupuncture.

AYURVEDA

Ayurveda, also referred to as *Ayurvedic medicine*, is a holistic system of medicine that was developed in ancient India and is now practiced primarily in the Indian sub-continent. Rather than addressing the symptoms of illness and disease, it focuses on helping patients to achieve and maintain balance of the mind, body, and spirit. In Ayurvedic medicine, a healthy person is one who has a clear mind, a calm and happy emotional state, and a body free of toxins because wastes have been properly eliminated.

According to Ayurveda, all objects in the universe including the human body are composed of five elements (earth, fire, water, air, and vacuum), which combine differently in individuals to create three *doshas*, or *life energies*. These are known as *Vata* (comprised of space and air), *Pitta* (comprised of fire and water), and *Kapha* (comprised of water and earth). Each dosha is associated with a certain body type and personality, and has a predisposition to certain health problems. Every person has his or her own balance of the three doshas, with one dosha being predominant. The doshas are believed to regulate every physiological and psychological process of man. When the doshas are in harmony, there is emotional balance and health. Symptoms of illness occur when the doshas are imbalanced. Imbalances may be caused by an unhealthy lifestyle or diet, improper mental or physical exertion, or exposure to environmental toxins.

In Ayurveda, diagnoses are made upon a holistic evaluation of the patient's physiological characteristics and mental disposition. Along with a general physical examination, the practitioner also checks for pulses (believed to be different for each dosha) and bodily sounds, examines feces and urine, and examines the tongue, eyes, and skin. Once a diagnosis is made, treatment involves many types of interventions that are designed to eliminate impurities in the body, reduce unpleasant symptoms, and improve peace and harmony in the patient. *Panchakarma* is an important part of Ayurvedic healing, and involves clearing the body of toxins through such interventions as vomiting, enemas, or fasting. Diet is also a very important part of Ayurveda. Special diets are frequently prescribed, along with the use of medicinal formulas that contain various natural substances including herbs, plant oils, spices, and in some cases metals and mineral substances. Because these "medicines" are not regulated in the same way that traditional foods and medicines are in the Western world, practitioners of conventional medicine worry that patients receiving Ayurvedic medical treatment could be exposed to certain health risks, including adverse interactions or even toxicity. Other types of intervention that are common in the practice of Ayurveda include yoga, massage, meditation, exercise, and psychotherapy.

Training in Ayurveda

In the United States, there is no formal process of certifying or training Ayurvedic medical practitioners, although some states have approved Ayurvedic schools. Many practitioners obtain their formal training in India, where training can lead to a bachelor's or doctoral degree in Ayurveda. Many practitioners who claim to offer Ayurvedic treatment have not been trained formally in a medical school, but have received training in only certain aspects of Ayurveda, such as massage or meditation. Therefore, it is important to ask questions about the practitioner's training before seeking Ayurvedic medicine.

Recommended resources for Ayurveda

Literature

Douillard, J. (2003) *Perfect Health for Kids: Ten Ayurvedic Health Secrets Every Parent Must Know.* Berkeley, CA: North Atlantic Books.

Frawley, D. (2003) *Ayurvedic Healing: A Comprehensive Guide.* India: Motlal Barnarsidass.

Hardy, M.L. (2001) 'Research in Ayurveda: Where do we go from here?' *Alternative Therapies in Health and Medicine, 7,* 2, 34–35.

Lad, V. (1985) *Ayurveda: The Science of Self-Healing.* Wilmot, WI: Lotus Press.

Lodha, R. and Bagga, A. (2000) 'Traditional Indian systems of medicine.' *Annals of the Academy of Medicine, Singapore, 29,* 1, 37–41.

Agencies, organizations, and websites

Ayurveda UK
PO Box 5761
Burton-on-Trent DE13 9YW, UK
Telephone: +44 (0)1283 815669
Website: www.ayurveda.uk.com
British organization offering courses, articles, and links relating to Ayurveda.

Department of Ayurveda, Yoga and Naturopathy, Unami, Sidda, and Homeopathy (AYUSH)
Government of India, IRCS Building 1 Red Cross Road
New Delhi 110001, India
Telephone: +91 (11) 2373 1758
Website: www.indianmedicine.nic.in
This is the Government of India's official site for Indian forms of medicine.

National Institute of Ayurvedic Medicine (NIAM)
584 Milltown Road
Brewster, NY 10509, USA
Telephone: +1 (845) 278-8700
Website: www.niam.com
This website offers extensive resources and information about Ayurveda. It is sponsored by Dr. Scott Gerson, who holds both a conventional medical degree and a PhD in Ayurveda from India.

HOMEOPATHY

Homeopathy (also called *homeopathic medicine*) was developed at the end of the 18th century by a German physician, Samuel Hahnemann, who was frustrated with the conventional medical practices of his time. He began a series of experiments called *provings*, which involved giving small doses of common remedies to healthy persons and observing the symptoms that occurred as a result of these experiments. In this way, he discovered that swallowing certain substances could produce symptoms that were similar to common medical conditions. This led to his development of a theory known as the *Law of Similars*, or "like cures like". The theory proposes that when a substance that causes medical symptoms is ingested in extremely small amounts, it can cure a medical condition that produces the same symptoms by stimulating the body's own healing mechanisms.

Treatment in homeopathy involves selecting homeopathic *remedies* that are matched not only to the patient's symptoms, but also to his or her lifestyle, overall constitution, and emotional state. Remedies are made from many types of substances. The majority are based on herbal or other plant substances, but many include minerals, animal substances (such as snake venom or cuttlefish ink), or even tiny amounts of drugs such as antibiotics. The remedies are extremely diluted, and may be taken in the form of tablets, liquids, powders, tinctures, or creams and ointments. When taken in liquid form, they are often diluted in alcohol. Homeopaths believe that the more diluted the remedy, the more effective the cure. For this reason, the remedies can be easily polluted by other substances. They must be stored in careful ways, and should not be taken in the presence of strong foods, tobacco or alcohol. Although most commonly used for medical illnesses, remedies do exist to treat the behavioral problems often associated with autism or attention deficit disorders. *Bach flower remedies*, discussed elsewhere in this book, are considered by some to be a subtype of homeopathic treatment and are commonly used for children with ADHD and learning disabilities.

Homeopathic remedies are generally considered to be safe because of the extreme dilution of the substances. However, some patients do report feeling worse for a brief time after starting a remedy. In the United States, homeopathic remedies are regulated by the Food and Drug Administration according to the same standards as non-prescription, over the counter drugs. They must meet certain standards of strength, purity, quality, and packaging which must include indications for use. In the United Kingdom there are five regulated homeo-pathic pharmacies. Because over the counter homeopathic remedies are widely available, many patients choose to self-medicate instead of seeking advice from a homeopathic physician.

Training in homeopathy

In the United States, training in homeopathy is offered through a variety of programs that may or may not lead to a diploma or certificate. Homeopathy is also part of the medical training in naturopathy. Three states (Connecticut, Arizona, and Nevada) license medical doctors specifically for homeopathy, while laws regulating practice vary in the other states. Most commonly, homeopathy is used as an adjunct to other medical practices in the United States.

In Europe, homeopathy training occurs as post-graduate training for doctors, or as a primary professional degree that takes from three to six years to complete.

Recommended resources for homeopathy

Literature

Chernin, D. (2006) *The Complete Homeopathic Resource for Common Illnesses.* Berkeley, CA: North Atlantic Books.

Cucherat, M., Haugh, M.C., Gooch, M. and Boissel, J.P. (2000) 'Evidence of clinical efficacy of homeopathy: A meta-analysis of clinical trials. Homeopathic Medicines Research Advisory Group.' *European Journal of Clinical Pharmacology, 56,* 1, 27–33.

Jacobs, J., Williams, A.L., Girard, C., Njike, V.Y. and Katz, D. (2005) 'Homeopathy for attention-deficit/hyperactivity disorder: A pilot randomized-controlled trial.' *Journal of Alternative and Complementary Medicine, 11,* 5, 799–806.

Jonas, W.B., Kaptchuk, T.J. and Linde, K.A. (2003) 'A critical overview of homeopathy.' *Annals of Internal Medicine, 138,* 5, 393–399.

Lee, A.C. and Kemper, K.J. (2000) 'Homeopathy and naturopathy: Practice characteristics and pediatric care.' *Archives of Pediatrics and Adolescent Medicine, 154,* 1, 75–80.

Speight, P. (1989) *Homeopathic Remedies for Children.* Saffron Walden, UK: C.W. Daniel Co. Ltd.

Ullman, D. (1992) *Homeopathic Medicine for Children and Infants.* New York: Tarcher Books.

Wells, H. (1994) *Homeopathy for Children: The Practical Family Guide.* Lanaham, MD: Element Books.

Agencies, organizations, and websites

British Homeopathic Association
Hahnemann House, 29 Park Street West
Luton LU1 3BE, UK
Telephone: +44 (0)870 444 3950
Website: www.trusthomeopathy.org

National Center for Homeopathy
801 N. Fairfax Street, Suite 306
Alexandria, VA 22314, USA
Telephone: +1 (877) 624-0613
Website: www.homeopathic.org
This is the leading United Sstates organization supporting and promoting
homeopathy.

Society of Homeopaths
11 Brookfield, Duncan Close, Moulton Park
Northampton NN3 6WL, UK
Telephone: +44 (0)845 450 6611
Website: www.homeopathy-soh.org
This is the largest organization registering homeopaths in the United Kingdom.

NATUROPATHY

Naturopathy (or *naturopathic medicine*) is a system of healing and health restoration
that is based upon the belief that given the right conditions, the human body has
an inherent ability to heal itself. Naturopaths believe that viruses and bacteria are
normally present in humans, and do not typically cause disease in a healthy
person. They believe that an unhealthy diet, inadequate exercise, and accumu-
lated body wastes weaken the body and allow disease to take hold. Treatment
focuses on cleansing and strengthening the body to support the natural healing
process. Diet is central to naturopathy, and remedies may include detoxification
through fasting, elimination diets to identify allergens, and recommendations
for adopting more healthful dietary practices. Most naturopaths take a holistic
approach to healing, and incorporate a variety of other modalities, such as light
therapy, hydrotherapy, herbalism, exercise, massage, acupuncture,
aromatherapy, and relaxation techniques. Most naturopaths prefer to avoid
medicines and surgery whenever possible in favor of more natural remedies.
They also believe strongly that prevention is more valuable than a cure, and for
that reason focus heavily on guiding patients to lead a healthy lifestyle.

Several systems of naturopathy exist. In India, naturopathy emphasizes
strict vegetarianism and yoga, along with other philosophies that differ from

Western forms of naturopathy. In the United States, there are two groups of practitioners that refer to themselves as naturopaths. *Naturopathic physicians* are trained in conventional medical sciences and are able to provide patients with complete medical care that incorporates both conventional and alternative interventions. When deemed appropriate, naturopathic physicians prescribe drugs and perform invasive procedures such as surgery, or refer to other medical specialists as necessary. The other group of practitioners who offer naturopathic services are called *traditional naturopaths*. These include people from a wide range of backgrounds who are not formally trained as medical practitioners. Their focus is on educating patients in the use of light, water, herbs, diet, and exercise to help to build a strong and healthy body in support of wellness.

Training in naturopathy

Several states in the United States and some Canadian provinces offer licensure as a naturopathic physician to students who graduate from a four-year nationally accredited naturopathic medical graduate school. After receiving a Doctor of Naturopathic Medicine (abbreviated ND or NMD) They must pass a state or provincial certification exam. Many naturopathic physicians have additional training in areas such as acupuncture or Chinese medicine. In the United Kingdom there are several programs that offer training in naturopathic medicine. Graduates from these programs are eligible for registration with the General Council and Register of Naturopaths.

Traditional naturopaths typically receive training from other practitioners or from correspondence courses, and their practice is not regulated.

Recommended resources for naturopathy

Literature

Lee, A.C. and Kemper, K.J. (2000) 'Homeopathy and naturopathy: Practice characteristics and pediatric care.' *Archives of Pediatric and Adolescent Medicine*, *154*, 1, 75–80.

Scott, J. and Scott, J. (1990) *Natural Medicine for Children*. London: Gaia Books, Ltd.

Smith, M.J. and Logan, A.C. (2002) 'Naturopathy.' *Medical Clinics of North America*, *86*, 1, 173–184.

Thiel, R.J. (2001) *Combining Old and New: Naturopathy for the 21st Century*. Warsaw, IN: Wendell W. Whitman Company.

Agencies, organizations, and websites

American Association of Naturopathic Physicians
4435 Wisconsin Avenue NW, Suite 403
Washington, DC 20016, USA
Telephone: +1 (866) 538-2267
Website: www.naturopathic.org
This organization offers publications and a directory of naturopathic practitioners in the United States.

American Naturopathic Certification Board
Website: www.acnb.net
This website offers information about continuing education opportunities, and provides certifications in two areas: CTN – Certified Traditional Naturopath, and CNW – Certified in Nutritional Wellness.

American Naturopathic Medical Accreditation Board
American Naturopathic Medical Association
PO Box 96273
Las Vegas, NV 89193, USA
Telephone: +1 (702) 897-7053
Website: www.anmab.org

Association of Naturopathic Practitioners
Coombe Hurst, Coombe Hill Road
East Grinstead, West Sussex RH19 4LZ, UK
Website: www.naturopathy-anp.com

National Institute of Naturopathy
Government of India, Ministry of Health and Family Welfare
Department of AYUSH, Bapu Bhavan, Tadiwala Road
Pune – 411 001, India
Telephone: +91 (20) 2605 9682
Website: www.punenin.org

The General Council and Registry of Naturopathy
Goswell House, 2 Goswell Road
Street BA16 0JG, UK
Telephone: +44 (0)870 7456 984
Website: www.naturopathy.org.uk
This is an independent registering body for naturopaths in the United Kingdom.

OSTEOPATHY

Osteopathy had its origins in the late 19th century. It was introduced by Andrew Still, a medical doctor, as an alternative approach to conventional (*allopathic*) medicine. Osteopathy is a holistic approach to intervention that emphasizes the role of the musculoskeletal system, including the bones, joints, muscles, ligaments, and connective tissues in health and disease. Osteopaths perform a variety of treatments that involve manipulative techniques. These may include stretching of soft tissue, passive joint movements, or high velocity thrust techniques, commonly referred to as *cracking*, to improve the range of motion within a joint. They believe that by treating various disorders of the musculoskeletal system, the body is better able to access its natural recuperative abilities.

The practice of osteopathy is very different in the United States than in other parts of the world. Internationally, osteopaths are considered a complementary therapy, and their treatments are largely limited to the manual treatment of musculoskeletal disorders, such as back, neck, or head pain, using similar techniques to those used in chiropractic intervention or in craniosacral therapy. In the United States, osteopathic physicians (DO) are medically trained physicians who have training that is considered the legal and professional equivalent of the Doctor of Medicine (MD) degree. They have the opportunity to train in all of the medical sub-specialty fields, and provide the full range of traditional medical interventions, including diagnosing disease, admitting to hospitals, prescribing drugs, and performing surgery. Osteopathic physicians in the United States are trained to perform physical or manual treatments (referred to as *osteopathic manual medicine*), including techniques that are used in chiropractic treatment or in craniosacral therapy. However, the use of these techniques by osteopathic physicians is not the predominant feature of their practice, and appears to be declining in popularity.

Training in osteopathy

Osteopathic medical schools represent approximately 16 percent of accredited medical schools in the United States. The training is comparable to that leading to a Doctor of Medicine degree, including two years of classroom-based instruction and two years of rotation through the various medical specialties. Following graduation, the physicians may opt to pursue specialty residency or fellowship programs. Osteopathic physicians must be licensed to practice in the state where they provide services.

In the United Kingdom, osteopathy has developed as a distinct profession. Osteopaths train in one of several institutions that are accredited by the General

Osteopathic Council. Graduates are then registered by this council. Most British osteopaths are not medically trained doctors, although some doctors choose to pursue osteopathic training as a post-graduate interest.

Recommended resources for osteopathy

Literature

Gevitz, N. (2004) *The DOs: Osteopathic Medicine in America.* Baltimore, MD: Johns Hopkins University Press.

Frymann, V.M., Carney, R.E. and Springall, P. (1992) 'Effect of osteopathic medical management on neurological development in children.' *Journal of the American Osteopathic Association, 92,* 6, 729–744.

Agencies, organizations, and websites

American Academy of Osteopathy
3500 DePauw Boulevard, Suite 1080
Indianapolis, IN 46268, USA
Telephone: +1 (317) 879-1881
Website: www.academyofosteopathy.org
The mission of this organization is to teach, advocate, and research the science, art, and philosophy of osteopathic medicine.

American Association of Colleges of Osteopathic Medicine
5550 Friendship Boulevard, Suite 310
Chevy Chase, MD 20815-7231, USA
Telephone: +1 (301) 968-4100
Website: www.aacom.org
This organization offers an on-line application service for all students applying to osteopathic medical schools in the United States. It also serves to advocate for research and public policy for the profession.

American Osteopathic Association
142 East Ontario Street
Chicago, IL 60611, USA
Telephone: +1 (800) 621-1773
Website: www.osteopathic.org
This is the professional organization for osteopathic physicians in the United States. It accredits osteopathic medical schools and certifies physicians.

British School of Osteopathy
275 Borough High Street
London SE1 1JE, UK
Telephone: +44 (0)207 089 5316 (student admission)
                +44 (0)207 089 5360 (clinic appointments)

Website: www.bso.ac.uk
This is the largest and oldest school of osteopathy in the United Kingdom.

General Osteopathic Council
176 Tower Bridge Road
London SE1 3LU, UK
Telephone: +44 (0)207 357 6655
Website: www.osteopathy.org.uk
This council serves to regulate the profession and ensure the quality of training.
It offers links to registered osteopaths throughout the United Kingdom.

Chapter 4

MIND-BODY INTERVENTIONS

ALERT PROGRAM

The *Alert Program* was designed to help children learn to self-regulate their level of alertness so that they can attend appropriately to a variety of situations or learning tasks. The program was developed by two occupational therapists, Mary Sue Williams and Sherry Shellenberger, and is based on principles combining sensory integration and cognitive theories of learning. Using the analogy of an automobile engine, children learn to recognize when their engine is going "too fast", "too slow" or "just right". They then learn to change their engine levels through various sensorimotor techniques such as putting something in their mouth (e.g. a hard candy to suck on or a water bottle), taking a motor break (such as getting up to sharpen a pencil), or touching something (such as a small toy to fidget with when listening). The techniques are adaptable for young children through adults, and are easily integrated into a whole classroom setting. Parents can also easily learn the language and techniques to use at home.

Training in the Alert Program

Parents, teachers, or therapists can learn this program through continuing education opportunities, most commonly a two-day conference that has been developed by the authors. Because the techniques are quite simple, one can also learn the program through reading the Leader's Guide that was developed by the authors.

Recommended resources for the Alert Program

Literature

Barnes, K., Schoenfeld, H., Garza, L., Johnson, D. and Tobias, L. (2005) 'Preliminary: Alert Program for boys' disturbances in the school setting.' *American Occupational Therapy Association School System Special Interest Section Quarterly*, *12*, 1–4.

Laurel, M. (2000) 'Bringing sensory integration home: A parent perspective on the Alert Program for self regulation.' *Autism/Asperger's Digest Magazine,* *March-April,* 14–15.

Shellenberger, S. and Williams, M. (2002) '"How does your engine run?": The Alert Program for self-regulation.' In A.G. Fisher, E.A. Murray, and A.C. Bundy (eds.) *Sensory Integration: Theory and Practice, 2nd edn* Philadelphia, PA: FA Davis: 342–345.

Williams, M.S. and Shellenberger, S. (1996) *How Does Your Engine Run? Leader's Guide to the Alert Program for Self-Regulation, Revised Edn.* Albuquerque, NM: Therapy Works, Inc.

Agencies, organizations, and websites
Therapy Works, Inc.
4901 Butte Place NW
Albuquerque, NM 87120, USA
Telephone: +1 (877) 897-3478
Website: www.alertprogram.com

ANIMAL ASSISTED THERAPY

Interactions with animals are believed to reduce stress, increase motivation and sense of well-being, promote positive interactions, and increase communication skills. For this reason, animals may be appropriately involved in a wide variety of teaching and healthcare applications. The use of animals as a therapeutic resource can be divided into several categories: *animal assisted activities (AAA),* which use animals to provide opportunities for motivation, education, or recreation; *animal assisted therapy (AAT),* which is goal-directed intervention directed by health or human service providers working within the scope of their profession; *resident animals (RA),* where animals live in a facility full time and participate in spontaneous or planned interactions with patients and staff; and *human animal support services (HASS),* where animals are trained to help their companion patients cope with the effects of a disability. AAA and AAT have been used widely with children with disabilities including autism and other learning disabilities. Taking care of an animal's needs (brushing, putting on collars and leashes, opening and closing pet carriers) can be a tool for improving fine motor skills. Also, because of the special bond that exists between many people and animals, the interaction may help to facilitate learning, communication, and socialization skills. Because many children relate to animals as peers, it is often easier to teach them how to read the animal's body language and to understand the animal's feelings than to teach them to emphathize with other humans. AAT has special considerations, and cannot be used if there are certain health concerns, such as asthma or allergies, or if the child's behaviors could result in injury to the child or the animal. When used in institutional settings, animals must be appropriately immunized and licensed, and may be subject to health screening tests to assure that humans are not exposed to diseases that could be carried in the animals. Professionals who wish to use animals should check with local officials to determine what, if any, regulations apply. Many different types of animals may be used in these programs, and are often selected according to their match to a patient's personality and individual needs. *Hippotherapy* uses horses to achieve therapeutic goals. *Dolphin-assisted therapy* uses dolphins for short-term therapy. These specialized areas of AAT are discussed elsewhere in this book.

Training in animal assisted therapy

AAAs are used by a wide variety of professionals including teachers, social service workers, therapists, psychologists, and others. There is no specific regulation for the use of animals used in the context of other interventions, other than rules and regulations governing the health and safety of patients, workers, and animals. No specific training is required before incorporating animals into practice, but degree programs are available through many colleges, and other continuing education programs exist for professionals who wish to learn more about the topic.

Recommended resources for animal assisted therapy

Literature

Arkow, P. (1998) *How to Start a 'Pet Therapy' Program: A Guidebook for Health Care Professionals.* Colorado Springs, CO: The Humane Society of the Pikes Peak Region.

Arkow, P. (2004) *Animal-Assisted Therapy and Activities: A Study, Resource Guide, and Bibliography for the Use of Companion Animals in Selected Therapies, 9th edn.* Stratford, NJ: Phil Arkow/!deas.

Ballarini, G. (2003) 'Pet therapy: Animals in human therapy.' *Acta Bio-Medica: Atenei Parmensis, 74*, 2, 97–100.

Delta Society (1999) *Standards of Practice for Animal-Assisted Activities and Therapy.* Renton, WA: Delta Society.

Fine, A. (ed.) (2000) *Handbook on Animal-Assisted Therapy: Theoretical Foundations and Guidelines for Practice.* San Diego, CA: Academic Press.

Pavlides, M. (2008) *Animal-Assisted Interventions for Individuals with Autism.* London: Jessica Kingsley Publishers.

Wells, D.L. (2007) 'Domestic dogs and human health: An overview.' *British Journal of Health Psychology, 12*, pt 1, 145–156.

Agencies, organizations, and websites

American Veterinary Medical Association
1931 North Meacham Road, Suite 100
Schaumberg, IL 60173, USA
Telephone: +1 (847) 925-8070
Website: www.avma.org
This organization offers guidelines for various uses of animals in therapy programs, as well as links to other references and organizations.

Delta Society
875 124th Avenue NE, Suite 101
Bellevue, WA 98005-2531, USA
Telephone: +1 (425) 679-5500
Website: www.deltasociety.org
Organization offering extensive information and resources relating to animals in therapy.

International Association of Human-Animal Interaction Organizations
SCAS-UK
10B Leny Road
Callander FK17 8BA, Scotland
Telephone: +44 (0)1877 330996
Website: www.iahaio.org

Phil Arkow/!deas
37 Hillside Road
Stratford, NJ 08084, USA
Telephone: +1 (856) 627-5118
Website: www.animaltherapy.net

Society for Companion Animal Studies
The Blue Cross, Shilton Road
Burford, Oxon OX18 4PF, UK
Telephone: +44 (0)1993 825597
Website: www.scas.org.uk
This society offers training in animal assisted therapy, supports research, and produces a number of publications.

APPLIED BEHAVIORAL ANALYSIS

Applied behavioral analysis (ABA) is an educational methodology widely used with children with autism and other severe learning disabilities. It is based on the principles of *operant conditioning* and involves systematically reinforcing desired behaviors through rewards which may include praise, tokens, or edibles, and discouraging undesired behaviors by ignoring or redirecting them. A basic principle of ABA is that every behavior has identifiable *antecedents* (events or environmental contexts leading up to the behavior), and results in a predictable *consequence* (outcome of the behavior). By carefully analyzing what antecedents lead to a particular behavior, and then providing a consistent consequence to that behavior that is based on the person's individual preferences, the behavior may be gradually shaped into one that is more desirable. ABA is commonly used by behavioral psychologists to address such problems as reducing self-injurious behavior or treating severe eating disorders. For children with autism, ABA has gained popularity primarily due to the work of Dr O. Ivor Lovaas, a professor of psychology based at the University of California at Los Angeles. Lovaas developed a particular approach to ABA which is used primarily to teach communication skills and to reduce certain behaviors, especially tantrums and acting out behaviors, in young children with autism. His approach involves the use of *discrete trials*, which are a series of distinct, repetitive lessons targeting a specific behavior (for example, looking at the speaker when the word "hello" is said, or pointing to the correct picture when asked, "Show me the dog."). Each trial consists of a request for the child to perform an action, followed by a specific reaction or consequence depending on whether the child correctly performed the task. Correct behaviors are initially rewarded with a token or food reward, but rewards are gradually phased out and are replaced with more natural consequences, such as praise or a hug. Trials are repeated every three to five seconds until the behavior is learned. Lovaas and his followers recommend that this type of therapy be introduced at an early age, preferably by two years of age and no later than six years of age. The intervention is extremely intensive, requiring approximately 30 to 40 hours per week of one-on-one training for a continuous period of two to three years. Because of its intensity, the program may require multiple trainers who must strictly adhere to the exact same protocol for each trial. *Discrete trial therapy*, or *Lovaas therapy* refers to applied behavior analysis that is conducted using the specific techniques and protocols as developed by Dr Lovaas, but other types of ABA may also be used with children who have autism.

In recent years, another model that is based upon ABA principles has emerged and is gaining in popularity. The *Verbal Behavior (VB)* approach is based upon theories of verbal language development that were introduced by psychologist B.F. Skinner in the 1950s. Skinner disputed the prevailing notion that language represents an innate biological or cognitive ability that develops naturally and according to a predictable developmental sequence. Instead, he argued that language develops in response to specific environmental challenges, and that communicative efforts are encouraged, rewarded, punished, extinguished, or ignored depending on the environmental context, as the child attempts to become a full member of a verbal community. He developed an analysis of verbal behavior that focuses on the *function* of words, as opposed to the *meaning* of words. During the 1980s, several psychologists built upon Skinner's analysis to develop the verbal behavioral approach. Like Lovaas' approach, VB incorporates the principles of applied behavioral analysis. However, there are several distinct differences between the two approaches. First, the Lovaas approach assumes that receptive language precedes expressive language, while VB focuses on teaching specific components of expressive language and on increasing the child's motivation to communicate verbally. In Lovaas training, the therapist selects what words will be taught, and assumes that the child has learned the word when he or she can correctly point to the object or picture when the therapist says, for example, "Show me the ball." In the VB approach, intervention begins with teaching the child to request desired objects, information, or activities, referred to as *mand training*. This concept builds on the child's inner drive and motivation to obtain things that he or she wants. During mand training, children are taught to understand the multiple functions of words and language, and to use those words spontaneously in naturally occurring contexts. If, for example, the child enjoys playing with balls, he or she must demonstrate an understanding of multiple meanings and uses of the word "ball" before it is considered mastered. The child must be able to ask for a ball, and find one when prompted to do so. When presented with a selection of toys including a ball, he or she must also correctly respond when asked questions like, "What do you like to play with?", "Give me something round," "Tell me your favorite toy." The child must also be able to answer questions about the ball when it is out of sight, for example, "What bounces?" Another distinguishing feature of the VB approach is that training is planned to occur in the natural environment. This is something that is not typical of the more structured Lovaas training, and may help to promote better generalization of skills that are learned through discrete trials.

There is a fair amount of scientific evidence to support the effectiveness of ABA techniques as a valid scientific intervention for children with autism. Lovaas first published a study in 1987 suggesting that close to half of the children treated using his specific protocol gained "normal" functioning and could be educated in mainstream settings. Replication studies continue to support the claims of Lovaas. Critics, however, suggest that these studies select subjects that are not representative of the autism population at large, and that the gains are not likely to be as large as predicted. Criticism is also heard about the intensity and cost of the program, as well as concern that it teaches "splinter" skills that will not generalize to other behaviors. Previously, some Lovaas programmes included the use of aversive reinforcers, such as slapping the child, as a punishment for negative behaviors. Although the use of aversive reinforcement is no longer endorsed by most followers of Lovaas, parents are cautioned that some individual practitioners may include aversives as part of the program. There is more limited empirical evidence to support the effectiveness of the VB approach. Although preliminary studies are promising, there is no long-term outcome data for this approach.

Training in applied behavioral analysis

Professionals from a variety of fields, including psychologists, educators, social workers, occupational therapists, speech-language therapists, and medical specialists, are exposed to the principles of applied behavior analysis as part of their entry-level professional education. These professionals must meet regulatory standards as established by their profession. Advanced training is available through a number of continuing education programs. The Behavior Analyst Certification Board®, based in the United States, offers two levels of certification for practitioners interested in specializing in ABA. Certification is granted upon the completion of required courses and successful passing of an exam. Certification is based in the United States, but is available to practitioners who have trained in other countries, as long as they meet the basic United States standards. Practitioners with a minimum of a Bachelor's degree may become Board Certified Associate Analysts (BCABA) and are trained to carry out specific behavior interventions. Practitioners with a minimum of a Master's degree may become Board Certified Behavior Analysts (BCBA) and may design and implement programs, as well as supervising Associate Behavior Analysts.

Recommended resources for applied behavioral analysis

Literature

Anderson, M. (2007) *Tales From the Table: Lovaas/ABA Intervention with Children on the Autism Spectrum*. London: Jessica Kingsley Publishers.

Barbera, M.L. and Rasmussen, T. (2007) *The Verbal Behavior Approach: How to Teach Children with Autism and Related Disorders*. London: Jessica Kingsley Publishers.

Carr, J.E. and Firth, A.M. (2005) 'The Verbal Behavior Approach to early and intensive behavioral intervention for autism: A call for additional empirical support.' *Journal of Early and Intensive Behavioral Intervention, 2*, 1, 18–27.

Cohen, H., Amervine-Dickens, M. and Smith, T. (2006) 'Early intensive behavioral treatment: Replication of the UCLA model in a community setting.' *Journal of Developmental and Behavioral Pediatrics, 27*, 2 supplement, 145–155.

Greer, R.D. and Ross, D.E. (2007) *Verbal Behavior Analysis: Inducing and Expanding New Verbal Capabilities in Children with Language Delays*. Upper Sadle River, NJ: Allyn and Bacon.

Lovaas, O.I. (1987) 'Behavioral treatment and normal educational and intellectual functioning in young autistic children.' *Journal of Consulting and Clinical Psychology, 55*, 1, 3–9.

Lovaas, O.I. (2003) *Teaching Individuals with Developmental Delays: Basic Intervention Techniques*. Austin, TX: Pro-Ed.

Lovaas, O.I. and Smith, T. (2003) 'Early and intensive behavioral intervention in autism.' In A.E. Kazdin and J.R. Weisz (eds.) *Evidence-Based Psychotherapies for Children and Adolescents* (pp. 325–340). New York: Guilford Press.

Richman, S. (2001) *Raising a Child with Autism: A Guide to Applied Behavior Analysis for Parents*. London: Jessica Kingsley Publishers.

Sallows, G.O. and Graupner, T.D. (2005) 'Intensive behavioral treatment for children with autism: Four year outcome and predictors.' *American Journal of Mental Retardation, 110*, 6, 417–438.

Shea, V. (2004) 'A perspective on the research literature related to early intensive behavioral intervention (Lovaas) for young children with autism.' *Autism, 8*, 4, 349–367.

Skinner, B.F. (1957) *Verbal Behavior*. Acton, MA: Copley Publishers.

Sundberg, M.L. and Michael, J. (2001) 'The benefits of Skinner's analysis of verbal behavior for children with autism.' *Behavior Modification, 25*, 698–724.

Troutman, A. and Troutman, A.C. (2005) *Applied Behavior Analysis for Teachers, 7th edn*. Upper Saddle River, NJ: Prentice-Hall.

Agencies, organizations, and websites

Association for Behavior Analysis International
1219 South Park Street
Kalamazoo, MI 49001, USA
Telephone: +1 (269) 492-9310
Website: www.abainternational.org
This is the primary professional organization for members with an interest in applied behavior analysis. It offers a range of member services, as well as links to internationally affiliated chapters.

Behavior Analyst Certification Board®, Inc.

Metro Building, Suite 102
1705 Metropolitcan Boulevard
Tallahassee, FL 32308-3796, USA
Website: www.bacb.com
The mission of this organization is to develop, promote, and implement a
national and international certification program for behavior analyst
practitioners. It provides a mechanism for practitioners to obtain certification,
and provides information to consumers about ABA and where to find certified
practitioners.

Lovaas Institute

East Headquarters:
52 Haddonfield-Berlin Road, Suite 1000
Cherry Hill, NJ 08034, USA
Telephone: +1 (856) 616-9442
West Headquarters:
11500 West Olympic Boulevard, Suite 318
Los Angeles, CA 90064, USA
Telephone: +1 (310) 914-5433
Website: www.lovaas.com
This is the official website for the Lovaas method of applied behavior analysis,
offering a range of information, links, and educational programs. It provides
clinic-based direct services in many cities in the United States, and provides
consultative services throughout the United States.

Parents for the Early Intervention of Autism in Children (PEACH)

The Brackens, London Road
Ascot, Berkshire SL5 8BE, UK
Telephone: +44 (0)1344 882248
Website: www.peach.org.uk
This is a parent-led charity devoted to promoting early behavioral intervention
to young children with autism using ABA.

UK Young Autism Project

Room 107, Mortlake High Street
London SW14 8JN, UK
Telephone: +44 (0)208 392 3931
Website: www.ukyap.org
This organization is a research-based replication program conducting outcome
studies as part of a multi-site Young Autism Project directed by Dr Lovaas and
Dr Tristam Smith at the University of California at Los Angeles. It provides
center-based services in Bristol, Birmingham, and London, and can provide
consultative services elsewhere in the United Kingdom.

AROMATHERAPY

Aromatherapy refers to the selected, therapeutic use of essential plant oils to improve health and well-being. It is thought to be one of the oldest forms of holistic medicine, originating in Egypt more than 5000 years ago. Often combined with massage, aromatherapy is believed to have influence upon several primitive parts of the brain that are associated with emotional regulation. For example, peppermint oil is believed to be stimulating to the nervous system, and may help to improve concentration. Using a variety of techniques, pure essential oils are extracted from plant materials and are combined with a carrier oil for use in therapy. These oils tend to be costly due to the enormous volume of plant material required to produce even a small amount of essential oil, and because of the complexity of extraction techniques. Because the cost of true essential oil may seem prohibitive, many synthetic fragrances have been developed that mimic the fragrance of essential oils. Unfortunately, however, synthetic fragrances are believed to lack therapeutic value. Peppermint candies or food flavoring will therefore not produce the same therapeutic effect as pure essential peppermint oil. Aromatherapists are taught to understand the chemistry of essential oils, and learn to formulate mixtures that produce desired health or emotional benefits. Most oils are considered to fall into one of four categories: stimulating, sedative, regulating, or euphoric. Aromatherapy is an intervention that has been widely used to reduce stress and promote improved attention and coping among children with autism spectrum disorders and other learning disabilities. Application can take several forms including: scented cotton or beads for inhalation purposes, use of a diffuser or adding oils to baths, or combining with therapeutic massage. The use of aroma alone is believed to affect the brain directly, while using oils with a bath or massage allows the oils to be absorbed by the skin to work internally. Aromatherapy is usually considered to be a fairly safe intervention, but there is the potential for side effects, especially related to allergies or to skin reactions. Also, oils are flammable and subject to chemical changes, and therefore require special storage precautions. The use of aromatherapy as an adjunctive therapy tends to be more widely accepted in the United Kingdom than in the United States.

Training in aromatherapy

Currently, in the United States there is no official regulation of aromatherapy nor of the essential oils. Many schools offer training that leads to a diploma or certificate of training, but there is no official accreditation of these schools. Because some states require certification or licensure in a professional field before one can lay hands on a patient, aromatherapy is often incorporated into the practice of a professional nurse, massage therapist, occupational therapist, or other health care provider.

In the United Kingdom, there are a number of diploma courses that allow one to obtain insurance and to practice as an aromatherapist. Further training allows one to meet national standards and to become a registered aromatherapist.

Recommended resources for aromatherapy

Literature

Devereaux, C. (2002) *Aromatherapy Essential Oils and How to Use Them.* London: Edison Sadd.

Hudson-Maxwell, C. (1994) *Aromatherapy Massage: The Complete Guide to Massaging with Essential Oils.* New York: D.K. Publishing.

Patricia, M. (2004) 'Complementary therapies for children: Aromatherapy.' *Paediatric Nursing, 16*, 7, 28–30.

Price, S. and Price, L. (1999) *Aromatherapy for Health Professionals, 2nd edn.* London: Churchill Livingstone.

Schnaubelt, M. (1999) *Medical Aromatherapy: Healing with Professional Oils.* Berkeley, CA: Frog Ltd.

Tisserand, R. (1999) *The Art of Aromatherapy, 19th edn.* Saffron Walden, UK: The C.W. Daniel Company Ltd.

Williams, T.I. (2006) 'Evaluating effects of aromatherapy massage on sleep in children with autism: A pilot study.' *Evidence Based Complementary and Alternative Medicine, 3*, 3, 373–377.

Agencies, organizations, and websites

Aromatherapy Council
PO Box 6522
Desborough, Kettering, Northants NN14 2YX, UK
Telephone: +44 (0)870 7743 477
Website: www.aromatherapycouncil.co.uk
Website offers information about schools and the registration process, and provides a comprehensive listing of member associations in the United Kingdom.

Aromatherapy Registration Council™
C/-5940SW Hood Ave
Portland, OR 97039, USA
Telephone: +1 (503) 244 0726

Website: www.aromatherapycouncil.org
This is a non-profit organization in the United States that offers voluntary, periodic registration that includes an examination for aromatherapists who have completed certain educational requirements.

International Federation of Aromatherapists (IFA)
62–63 Churchfield Road
London W3 6AY, UK
Telephone: +44 (0)208 992 9605
Website: www.ifaroma.org
The oldest established organization for professional aromatherapists in the world.

National Association for Holistic Aromatherapy
3327 W. Indian Trail Road PMB 144
Spokane, WA 99208, USA
Telephone: +1 (508) 325-3419
Website: www.naha.org

ART THERAPY

Art therapy is a form of psychotherapy that utilizes art materials and the creative process to improve the physical, mental, and emotional well-being of individuals. Through the process of creative expression, patients are able to more fully express their feelings and emotions. It is a therapy that is especially effective for children, who tend to have more difficulty than adults when expressing themselves using words. Talent is not necessary for therapy to be effective. However, art therapy may be especially appealing to children with autism spectrum disorders because they often possess a natural talent for the arts. Often, children's drawings are used as an assessment tool, as the hidden meaning in the drawings can offer the therapist clues as to the child's issues and concerns. As the child is guided to talk about his or her art, the therapist can help the child to externalize thoughts, experiences and feelings. Often, this produces less anxiety than simply talking about feelings, as in more traditional counseling techniques.

Training in art therapy

Art therapists have a Master's degree in art therapy or a related field, and have specific training in counseling and psychotherapy as well as in the theory, methods, and practice of art therapy. While many types of practitioners incorporate art mediums into their therapeutic programs, professional art therapists must meet rigorous requirements for training and supervision in order to meet registration requirements. In the United States, art therapists may become registered through the Art Therapy Credentials Board, and use the initials ATR to indicate registration. In the United Kingdom, practice is regulated through the Health Professions Council.

Recommended resources for art therapy

Literature

Edwards, D. (2004) *Art Therapy. Creative Therapies in Practice Series.* London: Sage Publications.

Evans, K. and Dubowski, J. (2001) *Art Therapy with Children on the Autism Spectrum: Beyond Words.* London: Jessica Kingsley Publishers.

Pratt, R.R. (2004) 'Art, dance, and music therapy.' *Physical Medicine and Rehabilitation Clinics of North America, 15*, 4, 827–841.

Waller, D. (2006) 'Art therapy for children: How it leads to change.' *Clinics in Child Psychology and Psychiatry, 11*, 2, 271–282.

Agencies, organizations, and websites

American Art Therapy Association, Inc.
5999 Stevenson Avenue
Alexandria, VA 22304, USA
Telephone: +1 (888) 290-0878
Website: www.arttherapy.org
This is an American organization of professionals involved in art therapy, and offers a range of information, publications, and educational opportunities.

Art Therapy Credentials Board
3 Terrace Way, Suite B
Greensboro, NC 27403-3660, USA
Telephone: +1 (877) 213-2822
Website: www.atcb.org
This American organization provides several options for registration as an art therapist, and provides a directory of qualified therapists.

British Association of Art Therapists
24–27 White Lion Street
London N1 9PD, UK
Telephone: +44 (0)207 686 4216
Website: www.baat.org
This is the professional organization for art therapists in England.

Health Professions Council
Park House, 184 Kennington Park Road
London SE11 4BU, UK

Telephone: +44 (0)207 582 0866

Website: www.hpc-uk.org

This is the regulatory agency for art therapists in the United Kingdom.

ASSISTIVE TECHNOLOGY FOR LITERACY SKILLS

In the past several decades, there has been tremendous growth in the available technologies to support students with disabilities in learning to read and write. However, educators and other professionals vary widely in their knowledge of, and experience with, applied technology. As a result, many students who might benefit from assistive technology are under identified, or are taught using technology that is familiar to the educator but might not be the best solution for an individual student. It is beyond the scope of this book to discuss the full range of possibilities; however, some of the more common applications will be summarized.

Assistive technology refers to any tool or device that makes the child more independent in learning tasks. It can be very simple (*low-tech*), such as highlighting important words in text, or very complicated (*high-tech*), such as converting printed text to synthesized speech.

Numerous software programs exist that encourage students to have practice and repetition in learning academic skills such as phonemic awareness, grammar, spelling, or number skills. Many programs offer enticing graphics, immediate positive feedback for successful responses, and the ability to track progress over time.

Some students with the specific learning disability known as *visual dyslexia* have difficulty staying focused on a word or a line of text, as the words appear to be shifting or moving around. Various magnifiers, such as the *visual tracking magnifier*, allow the student to run the magnifier over a word or line of print so that only a small section of text is magnified and brought to his or her attention. Colored overlays, color projecting lights, or highlighters can also serve to draw attention to important text and make viewing easier.

For students who have severe difficulty reading material from a book or a printed page, several options are available. Several organizations offer *recorded books*, but the selection of available books may be limited. When needed, computers can actually convert printed text from a book or magazine into synthesized speech that is read aloud on the computer. This requires a scanner, scanning software, *optical character recognition (OCR) software*, *text-to-speech software*, and a compatible computer. The *Kurzweil 3000 LearnStation* and *OmniPage® Pro 14* are examples of this type of software. For students who have the OCR and scanning software, there are a number of internet resources that offer public-domain books, stories, and articles that can be downloaded and scanned. Other software, such as *Write: OutLoud SOLO*™ allows text to be formatted so it is easier to read by highlighting certain text, changing color and font features, or pairing graphics with text. Students who can read most text but who struggle with decoding certain unfamiliar words may benefit from a *reading pen*, which allows the user to run the pen over the word, then hear both the pronunciation and a definition of the word.

For students who have difficulty writing, a number of assistive technology solutions are available. Special pencil grips, inclined writing boards, or paper with raised lines can help the physical task of writing. Most students with or without disabilities find it easier to write using a word processing program. Portable word processors, such as the *AlphaSmart® 3000* can be helpful when access to a full computer is impractical. Portable word processors offer many features that help struggling writers, such as spelling and grammar checks, autocorrect, and dictionary and thesaurus access. Students who have difficulty with vocabulary and word finding may benefit from *word prediction* software that displays a list of possible words after the student has typed in a few letters.

Specialized software is also available for students who have difficulty organizing their ideas to generate writing. Programs like *Kidspiration* or *Draftbuilder®* support the student in brainstorming ideas, developing an outline, and preparing a first draft for writing.

When writing problems are extreme, computers may be fitted with *speech recognition software* that allows the student to speak into a microphone while the words are translated into text on the computer.

Students with significant motor limitations that impact their ability to access a computer have many options for alternative access. Specialized mouses or other input devices such as touch windows are just a few of the possibilities that exist.

When choosing to use assistive technology, be sure that the technology matches the child's needs and that he or she is motivated to use the technology. Carefully consider the cost involved, and understand that technology may draw unwanted attention from others. It is also helpful to consider that some technologies lack portability and may therefore be useful only in selected settings.

Training in assistive technology

Professionals from a variety of disciplines, especially special educators, occupational therapists, physical therapists, and psychologists receive varying amounts of instruction in assistive technology practices during their routine professional training. Many colleges and universities offer advanced training through graduate programs in these disciplines. Additional training is available through independent study or participating in continuing education workshops. The Rehabilitation Engineering and Assistive Technology Society of North America (RESNA) offers several voluntary certification programs for professionals interested in assistive technology. Because there are continual changes and innovations in the technology available, it is important to make sure that the professional involved in recommending and supervising the use of assistive technology applications maintains current familiarity with new advances in the field.

Recommended resources for assistive technology

Literature

Alliance for Technology Access (2004) *Computer Resources for People with Disabilities: A Guide to Assistive Technologies, Tools, and Resources for People of All Ages (Computer Resources for People with Disabilities).* Alameda, CA: Hunter House.

Council for Exceptional Children (2005) *Universal Design for Learning: A Guide for Teachers and Education Professionals.* Upper Saddle River, NJ: Prentice Hall.

Koppenhaver, D.A., Hendrix, M.P. and Williams, A.R. (2007) 'Toward evidence-based literacy interventions for children with severe and multiple disabilities.' *Seminars in Speech and Language, 28*, 1, 79–89.

Long, T.M., Woolverton, M., Perry, D.F. and Thomas, M.J. (2007) "Training needs of pediatric occupational therapists in assistive technology." *American Journal of Occupational Therapy, 61*, 3, 345–354.

Rose, D.H. and Meyer, A. (2002) *Teaching Every Student in the Digital Age: Universal Design for Learning.* Alexandria, VA: Association for Supervision and Curriculum Development.

Thompson, J.R., Bakken, J.P., Fulk, B.M. and Peterson-Karlan, G. (2004) *Using Technology to Improve the Literacy Skills of Students with Disabilities.* Available at www.ic-online.co.uk/dyslexia/page2/htm, accessed 26 June 2007.

Agencies, organizations, and websites

Ability Net
Telephone: +44 (0)1926 312847
Website: www.abilitynet.org.uk
With centres throughout the United Kingdom, this registered charity offers training, advice, technical assistance, and an on-line shop. The website offers links to its centers throughout the various regions of the United Kingdom.

ABLEDATA
8630 Fenton Street, Suite 930
Silver Spring, MD 20910, USA
Telephone: +1 (800) 227-0216
Website: www.abledata.com
Funded by the National Institute on Disability and Rehabilitation Research through the United States Department of Education, this is the largest available database for assistive technology equipment and related materials.

Alliance for Technology Access
1304 Southpoint Boulevard, Suite 240
Petaluma, CA 94954, USA
Telephone: +1 (707) 778-3011
Website: www.ataccess.org
This is an organization that focuses solely on technology for people with disabilities. It offers direct access to experts in assistive technology, training, technical assistance, and links to technology centers throughout the United States, where parents and professionals can explore and experiment with technology options.

Rehabilitation Engineering and Assistive Technology Society of North America (RESNA)
1700 N. Moore Street, Suite 1540
Arlington, VA 22209-1903, USA
Telephone: +1 (703) 524-6686
Website: www.resna.org
This is an interdisciplinary organization of professionals that promotes research, development, education, advocacy, and provision of technology. It offers voluntary certifications as an Assistive Technology Practitioner (ATP), Assistive Technology Supplier (ATS), or Rehabilitation Engineering Technician (RET).

AUDITORY TRAINING

A number of *auditory training* programs have been developed to address the needs of children and adults who have *central auditory processing disorders* as the result of developmental disabilities including autism, ADHD, and learning disabilities. Each of these programs involves having the patient wear headphones and listen to music that has been electronically altered in such a way as to train the auditory system to listen more selectively and to process auditory information without distortion or hypersensitivity. *Auditory Integration Training (AIT)* is the most widely used and researched of these methods, and will be discussed in this section. However, a number of other methods are also popular.

AIT refers to the system of therapy based on the original work of Guy Berard, an Ear-Nose-and-Throat specialist who introduced this intervention in France in the 1960s, and in the United States in 1991. Therapy based strictly upon his principles is known by several terms, including AIT, Berard Method, and *Digital Auditory Aerobics (DAA)*. Designed for children over the age of three, AIT is based upon the theory that children with developmental disabilities, including autism, ADHD, and other learning disabilities, often experience sensory processing difficulties that include hypersensitivity to sounds or hearing distortions. In the diagnostic phase of AIT, a detailed audiological evaluation is conducted, which looks at the patient's hearing in ranges that are wider than those used for traditional hearing tests. The results are examined to determine whether there is heightened awareness of particular frequencies which may relate to the patient's history of sound sensitivities or behavioral patterns, or whether there are significant discrepancies in sensitivity between the two ears. If the patient is considered to be an appropriate candidate for the training, the treatment consists of wearing earphones and listening to music that has been computer-modified by reducing the predictability of auditory patterns, and removing frequencies that cause sensitivity. Proponents claim that for treatment to be effective, there must be strict adherence to a protocol that involves twenty half-hour sessions, twice daily for ten days, with a minimum of 3½ hours between the daily sessions. Treatment is usually concluded at the end of ten days, but may be repeated after an interval of 9 to 12 months for some patients. Reported results include improved attention and listening skills, improved language and auditory comprehension, and behavioral changes including reduced lethargy and irritability. However, there is limited scientific evidence to support these claims, and the intervention is considered to be controversial within the medical community.

Some other popular systems of auditory training that are used for children with developmental disorders include the *Tomatis Listening Therapy Method*, *SAMONAS (Spectral Activated Music of Optimal Natural Structure)*, *The Listening Program*, and the *Dynamic Listening System*. These methods have not been subjected to scientific review as extensively as AIT, and the results claimed by advocates of these methods are therefore based upon more limited research combined with anecdotal report.

Training in auditory training

The use of various methods of auditory training is not formally regulated in either the United States or the United Kingdom, but is recognized as a controversial treatment that may be incorporated into the practice of many professionals, including occupational therapists, speech-language therapists, audiologists, psychologists, physicians, and special educators. Training generally consists of attendance at professional seminars, with certificates of completion or registration occurring as a result of completing case studies or signing agreements to practice the method using specific instruments and protocols as endorsed by the particular agency.

Recommended resources for auditory training

Literature

American Academy of Pediatrics Committee on Children with Disabilities (1997) 'Auditory integration therapy and facilitated communication for autism.' *Pediatrics, 102,* 431–433.

Berard, G. (1993) *Hearing Equals Behavior.* New Canaan, CT: Keats Publishing, Inc.

Bettison, S. (1996) 'The long-term effects of auditory training on children with autism.' *Journal of Autism and Developmental Disorders, 26,* 3, 361–374.

Brown, M.M. (1999) 'Auditory integration training and autism: Two case studies.' *British Journal of Occupational Therapy, 62,* 1, 13–18.

Cummings, R.L. (1986) 'An evaluation of the Tomatis listening training program.' *Dissertation Abstracts International, 47,* 858–859.

Sinha, Y., Silove, N., Wheeler, D. and Williams, K. (2006) 'Auditory integration training and other sound therapies for autism spectrum disorders: A systematic review.' *Archives of Disease in Childhood, 91,* 12, 1018–1022.

Agencies, organizations, and websites

Advanced Brain Technologies
The Listening Program, 5748 South Adams Avenue Parkway
Ogden, UT 84405, USA
Telephone: +1 (801) 622-5676
Website: www.advancedbrain.com
This organization offers a different approach to listening therapy systems, including its own version of equipment and professional training programs.

Berard AIT Website
Website: www.berardaitwebsite.com
This is the official Berard website in the United States, and offers extensive resources relating to the intervention.

Berard Auditory Integration Systems, Inc.
690 Boyd Road
Leicester, NC 28748, USA
Telephone: +1 (828) 683-6900
7 Tokeneke Road
Darien, CT 06820, USA
Telephone: +1 (203) 655-1091
Website: www.auditoryintegration.net
These agencies offer Berard auditory integration training in the United States through center-based direct services, and through in-home programs for patients who are unable to travel to one of the two centers.

Dynamic Listening Systems, Inc.
5655 S. Yosemite Street, Suite 303
Greenwood, CO 80111, USA
Telephone: +1 (303) 320-5502
Website: www.dynamiclistening.com
This organization sponsors services and professional seminars for a Tomatis-based approach to listening therapy.

IDEA Training Center
20 Washington Avenue, Suite 108
North Haven, CT 06473, USA
Telephone: +1 (203) 234-7401
Website: www.ideatrainingcenter.com
This agency sponsors training seminars in Berard Auditory Integration Training.

Samonas Auditory Intervention
3435 Camino Del Rio South, Suite 336
San Diego, CA 92108, USA
Telephone: +1 (800) 726-6627 (US)
            +49 (0) 2381 98222 16 (Europe)
Generic email: info@samonas.com
Website: www.samonas.com
This is the organization that offers information and professional training in Samonas.

The Georgiana Institute
PO Box 10
Roxbury, CT 06783, USA
Telephone: +1 (860) 355-1545
Website: www.georgianainstitute.org
This organization is devoted to educating the public worldwide about the benefits of auditory integration therapy.

Tomatis Développement SA
25 Grand-Rue
L-1661 Luxembourg, France
Telephone: +33 (352) 262720
Website: www.tomatis-group.com
This is the official website for promoting the use of Tomatis training, including a listing of certified Tomatis centers throughout the world.

COLORED LENSES AND OVERLAYS

This intervention was developed by a school psychologist, Helen Irlen, during the early 1980s, after she observed that many individuals with reading problems expressed similar complaints of visual distortions, sensitivity to glare, headaches, and tired eyes, and that these complaints were most problematic when attempting to read black print on white paper. Irlen proposed that some individuals with reading disabilities suffer from a condition in which the retina of the eye is overly sensitive to certain frequencies of light. This condition, which she coined *scotopic sensitivity syndrome*, causes visual information to the brain to be distorted and easily misunderstood. Using a specialized machine called an *Intuitive Colorimeter* to determine an individual's color preference, the method involves prescribing colored lenses or vinyl overlays to filter out the light frequencies that cause distortion, and to reduce glare. Up to 7000 different tints are available, depending upon the individual's unique sensitivities. Often, the particular tint is chosen through trial and error. Proponents claim that for people affected with scotopic sensitivity syndrome, use of the colored glasses, contact lenses, or reading overlays can increase the speed of reading and reduce eyestrain. *ChromaGen*™ lenses are soft contact lenses that have a tiny, almost invisible speck of color that has been selected through assessment with the Intuitive Colorimeter. Use of these lenses allows the patient to benefit from the tint throughout his or her day.

Training in colored lenses and overlays

A two-day Irlen screener training workshop is offered by the Irlen Institute for professionals who are trained in education, psychology, or speech or occupational therapy. Prescription of tinted glasses or contact lenses must be done through a qualified vision specialist (optometrist or ophthalmologist) who will also assure that the child's vision is evaluated for other possible problems.

Recommended resources for colored lenses and overlays

Literature

Irlen, H. (1991) *Reading by the Colors: Overcoming Dyslexia and Other Disabilities through the Irlen Method.* Garden City Park, NY: Avery.

Menacker, S.J., Breton, M.E., Breton, M.L., Radcliffe, J. and Cole, G.A. (1993) 'Do tinted lenses improve the reading performance of dyslexic children?' *Archives of Ophthalmology, 111*, 213–218.

Noble, J., Orton, M., Irlen, S. and Robinson, G. (2004) 'A controlled field study of the use of coloured overlays on reading achievement.' *Australian Journal of Learning Disabilities, 9*, 2, 11–22.

Whiteley, H.E. and Smith, C.D. (2001) 'The use of tinted lenses to alleviate reading difficulties.' *Journal of Research in Reading, 24*, 1, 30–40.

Agencies, organizations, and websites

Cantor & Nissel Ltd
Market Place
Brackley, Northamptonshire NN13 7NN, UK
Telephone: +44 (0)1280 702002
Website: www.cantor-nissel.co.uk
This is a British distributor of ChromaGen™ contact lenses.

Cerium Visual Technologies, Ltd
Cerium Group Headquarters, Cerium Technology Park
Tenterden, Kent TN30 7DE, UK
Telephone: +44 (0)1580 765211
Website: www.ceriumvistech.co.uk
This company developed and manufactures the Intuitive Colorimeter used to determine the appropriate tints for an individual's needs. It sells other products, including a screening kit, colored overlays, and tinted lenses. It offers a worldwide listing of practitioners trained to use this technology.

ChromaGen™ USA Inc.
The Atrium at Rae Park, 8 John Walsh Boulevard
Peekskill, NY 10566, USA
Website:www.chromagen.us
This is the United States distributor for ChromaGen™ contact lenses.

Irlen Institute
5380 Village Road
Long Beach, CA 90808, USA
Telephone: +1 (800) 554-7536
Websites: www.irlen.com; www.irlenuk.com

DANCE MOVEMENT THERAPY

Dance/Movement therapy, sometimes referred to as *dance therapy* or *choreotherapy*, is the psychotherapeutic use of movement and dance to promote social, cognitive, emotional, and physical development. As a profession, dance therapy began in the 1940s with the work of Marian Chace, an American dancer who discovered that she could help patients with emotional disturbances to express their emotions through dance and movement. It is widely used with people who have serious emotional disturbances, but may also be helpful for children with developmental disabilities, including autism. Therapy can be provided through individual or group sessions. There are several approaches in dance therapy, but therapists commonly use techniques derived from the methods of psychoanalysis as proposed by psychiatrist Dr Carl Jung, in which a patient works with recurring images in his or her thoughts to derive meaning in life. Rather than teaching specific dance moves, the therapist instructs the patient to move whenever he or she feels the inner impulse to move. The therapist serves as a non-critical witness of the patient's movements. Following the session, the patient and therapist talk about the meaning of the movements, and the emotions that were expressed.

Training in dance movement therapy

Entry into the profession of dance movement therapy is at the Master's level. In the United States, The American Dance Therapy Association offers two levels of certification. Dance Therapist Registered (DTR) indicates a therapist trained at the Master's level in an approved program. A therapist with this designation is qualified to work in a professional setting as part of a team operating under professional supervision. Therapists who meet additional training requirements belong to the Academy of Dance Therapists Registered (ADTR), and are fully qualified to teach, to provide supervision, or to engage in private practice. In the United Kingdom, several universities offer professional training in dance movement therapy.

Recommended resources for dance movement therapy

Literature

Erfer, T. (1995) 'Treating children with autism in a public school system.' In F. Levy (ed.), *Dance and Other Expressive Arts Therapies*. New York: Routledge.

Koch, S. and Bräuninger, I. (2006) *Advances in Dance/Movement Therapy: Theoretical Perspectives and Empirical Findings*. Berlin: Logos.

Lee. S.B., Kim, J., Lee, S.H. and Lee, H.S. (2002) 'Encouraging social skills through dance: An inclusion program in Korea.' *Teaching Exceptional Children*, *35*, 5, 40–44.

Parteli, L. (1995) 'Aesthetic listening: Contributions of dance/movement therapy to the psychic understanding of motor stereotypies and distortions in autism and psychosis in children and adolescents. Special Edition: European Consortium for Arts Therapy Education (ECArtE).' *The Arts in Psychotherapy*, *22*, 3, 241–247.

Payne, H. (2006) *Dance Movement Therapy: Theory, Research, and Practice, 2nd edn.* New York: Routledge.

Ritter, M. and Low, K.G. (1996) 'The effectiveness of dance/movement therapy.' *The Arts in Psychotherapy*, *23*, 3, 249–260.

Agencies, organizations, and websites

American Dance Therapy Association
2000 Century Plaza, Suite 108, 10632 Little Patuxent Parkway
Columbia, MD 21044, USA
Telephone: +1 (410) 997-4040
Website: www.adta.org
This organization focuses on establishing and maintaining high standards of professional education and competence in the field of dance movement therapy. It offers a certification process for therapists to become DTR or ADTR.

The Association for Dance Movement Therapy UK
32 Meadfoot Lane
Torquay TQ1 2BW, UK
Telephone: +44 (0)1670 825140
Website: www.admt.org.uk
This is the professional organization for dance movement therapy in the United Kingdom, and provides links to several university programs offering graduate level training in dance movement therapy.

DAVIS DYSLEXIA CORRECTION® METHOD

The *Davis Dyslexia Correction® Method* was developed by an engineer and self-diagnosed dyslexic, Ron Davis, in the early 1980s. Davis claims that he was able to correct his own severe dyslexia by discovering a method to overcome the perceptual distortions that commonly occur in the condition. He theorized that dyslexia is the result of a perceptual talent, in which the dyslexic individual thinks through mental or visual imagery rather than using words or internal dialogue in the mind. Unlike people who reason through verbal strategies, which are linear and sequential in nature, people with dyslexia tend to use global logic and reasoning strategies. They tend to be artistic, creative, and good at solving practical problems, but struggle with word-based, linear, step-by-step reasoning. When *disoriented*, or confronted with an unfamiliar problem, they tend to look at the problem from multiple angles and perspectives, instead of systematically breaking down the problem into its successive steps.

This program involves working with a trained facilitator who first provides an assessment to determine if the child possesses the positive mental talents that are associated with dyslexia, and to identify areas of academic weakness. The next phase is called *orientation counseling*, and involves training the child to visualize objects from various positions using only his or her mind. This is referred to as *moving the mind's eye*. The child is taught to recognize and control the mental state that leads to perceptual distortions of letters, numbers, and words, and to "turn off" the thought processes that lead to these distortions so that he or she can return to a relaxed and focused state of mind. The next phase of training is called *symbol mastery*. This teaches the student to think using symbols and words. Using clay, the student creates models of letters, numbers, and punctuation marks to make sure they have an accurate perceptual reference for these symbols. Students next create clay models of *trigger words*, which are the short, abstract words such as "this", "and", or "the", which are hard for students with dyslexia to learn since they cannot form a logical mental picture to represent the word. Unlike other reading programs, the Davis method does not employ training in phonemic awareness, and does not incorporate repetition or drill, believing instead that learning will not be retained unless the student sees where the information fits into the "big picture". There is no literature to support Davis' theory of orientation and disorientation. In addition, scientific study of this method has yet to occur, although there is abundant anecdotal support for the method.

Training in the Davis Dyslexia Correction® Method

Professional training is available to teachers, counselors, and other professionals through the Davis Dyslexia Association International. Several introductory workshops are offered. In addition, a series of workshops and supervised clinical practicums lead to voluntary licensing as a facilitator of this method.

Recommended resources for the Davis Dyslexia Correction® Method

Literature

Davis, R.D. and Braun, E.M. (1997) *The Gift of Dyslexia: Why Some of the Smartest People Can't Read and How They Can Learn, Revised.* New York: The Berkley Publishing Group.

Agencies, organizations, and websites

Davis Dyslexia Association International
1601 Bayshore Highway, Suite 260
Burlinghame, CA 94010, USA
Telephone: +1 (610) 692-7141
Website: www.dyslexia.com
This website offers extensive information about the Davis Dyslexia Correction®
Method and related programs. It provides information about training
workshops and links to affiliates in other countries.

Davis Learning Foundation
PO Box 972
Canterbury, Kent CT1 9DN, UK
Telephone: +44 (0)1227 732288
Website: www.davislearningfoundation.org.uk
This is the affiliate organization for Britan and Ireland, and includes a listing of
licensed facilitators in the United Kingdom.

DIR®/FLOORTIME MODEL

DIR®/Floortime is a comprehensive framework for understanding and treating
children with autism and related disorders. It focuses on helping children to
relate, to think, and to communicate, instead of focusing on treating a set of
symptoms or problem behaviors. This framework was developed by Stanley
Greenspan, a child psychiatrist and specialist in autism, and his associate Serena
Wieder, who is a clinical psychologist and infant mental health expert. They
propose a comprehensive, interdisciplinary approach to help children with
autism develop skills in all areas, including social-emotional functioning, communication, thinking and learning, motor skills, body awareness, and attention.
The term DIR stands for the three components of this approach: *Developmental*,
which focuses on understanding the developmental milestones that every child
must master for healthy emotional and intellectual growth; *Individual-Difference*,
which refers to understanding the unique sensory processing differences in each
child, and how these differences impact learning and behavior; and *Relationship-Based*, which focuses on helping the child to form relationships with primary
caregivers and peers, and to teach others methods of interaction that will help to
foster development in the child with autism.

Central to this approach is an intensive home program, called *Floortime*, in
which parents and other helpers play with the child on his or her own developmental level, and gradually entice the child to interact and attend to play and to
social interactions. Floortime sessions last for approximately 20 minutes each,

and are usually prescribed for eight to ten times per day. Siblings, teachers, or therapists may engage in Floortime sessions along with parents, and teach them the subtle ways of breaking into the child's world. Because of the intensive nature of this approach, it is difficult for some families to find the necessary time to conduct the required Floortime sessions. However, proponents explain that Floortime is as much a philosophy of interaction as a defined intervention, and that the techniques, once learned, can be integrated into all aspects of the child's daily routine. Proponents also believe that the progress made is generally proportional to the amount of time that caregivers pull the child into Floortime interactions. Critics express concern about the amount of time that parents must devote to implementing this program, and about the lack of peer-reviewed published scientific research to support its effectiveness.

As a comprehensive intervention, the DIR®/Floortime model also incorporates intensive treatment sessions with other relevant professionals, especially occupational therapists who have advanced training in sensory integration therapy, and speech therapists who work on receptive and expressive language. Education in an integrated setting, where the child with autism must learn to communicate with typically developing peers, is also paramount to this approach.

Training in DIR®/Floortime

Professionals who have training and credentials in a variety of disciplines, including regular and special education, speech-language pathology, occupational therapy, physical therapy, developmental optometry, creative arts therapy, clinical social work, psychology, nursing, pediatrics, developmental pediatrics, child psychiatry, and infant mental health are eligible for training in the DIR®/Floortime method. A six-day program is available to enable licensed and credentialed professionals to incorporate DIR® principles and practices into their existing programs. An advanced certificate program, which requires attendance at two summer institutes, as well as the demonstration of advanced competencies, is also available.

Recommended resources for DIR®/Floortime
Literature
Greenspan, S.J. and Wieder, S. (2006) *Engaging Autism: Helping Children Relate, Communicate, and Think with the DIR Floortime Approach.* Cambridge, MA: Da Capo Press.

Wieder, S. and Greenspan, S.J. (2001) 'The DIR® (Developmental, Individual-Difference, Relationship-Based) approach to assessment and intervention planning.' *Bulletin of ZERO TO THREE, National Center for Infants, Toddlers, and Families, 21*, 4, 11–19.

Wieder, S. and Greenspan, S.J. (2003) 'Climbing the symbolic ladder in the DIR model through floor time/interactive play.' *Autism, 7*, 4, 425–435.

Wieder, S. and Greenspan, S.J. (2005) 'Can children with autism master the core deficits and become empathetic, creative and reflective? A ten to fifteen year follow-up of a subgroup of children with autism spectrum disorders (ASD) who received a comprehensive developmental, individual-difference, relationship-based (DIR) approach.' *The Journal of Developmental and Learning Disorders, 9*, 39–61.

Agencies, organizations, and websites

The Floortime Foundation
4938 Hampden Lane, Suite 229
Bethesda, MD 20814, USA
Website: www.floortime.org
This website offers an extensive discussion about the DIR®/Floortime model.

European DIR® Institute
Rino Noord-Holland, Liedseplein 5
1017 PR Amsterdam, The Netherlands
Telephone: +31 (0)20 625 08 03
Website: www.rino.nl
This institute is in the process of organizing DIR® training programs in the European Health Care System(s).

Interdisciplinary Council on Developmental and Learning Disorders (ICDL)
4938 Hampden Lane, Suite 800
Bethesda, MD 20814, USA
Telephone: +1 (301) 656-2667
Website: www.icdl.com
This Council was founded by Stanley Greenspan and Serena Wieder, who developed the DIR®/Floortime Model. It is the primary organization offering training in the model, and also has a directory of specialists who have completed the training.

DOLPHIN ASSISTED THERAPY

Dolphin assisted therapy is a method used to improve the physical, cognitive, and social-emotional behaviors of children with severe disabilities. It was first proposed as a therapeutic intervention during the 1960s and 1970s by several people, especially by Betsy Smith, who was an educational anthropologist, and by psychologist David Nathanson. In part due to media coverage, and to the almost universal appeal of the dolphins, it has gained increased popularity in recent years.

This therapy is offered throughout the world, generally in areas where dolphins live naturally, and can be provided using different protocols. Commonly, the child works with a person who is trained to facilitate interaction between the dolphin and the child. Goals are established according to the child's individual needs, and in many, but not all programs, the treatment is conducted by (or in conjunction with) a qualified speech, physical, or occupational therapist. Typically, the treatment is given for 40 minutes per day for 5 to 10 days. Part of the treatment involves having the child placed on a platform in the water while being encouraged to feed, play with, or otherwise interact with the dolphin. Some children are also allowed to swim with the dolphins, which is said to increase communication and social skills. Proponents believe that this therapy works because dolphins have a natural affinity towards humans, especially those with disabilities. As in other *animal assisted therapies*, the bond between animal and human serves to motivate behavioral changes in the child, and give him or her a "jump start" to achieving therapy goals. Some proponents also believe that the sounds made by the *echolocation* system of communication in dolphins has the ability to modify human brain waves, helping to promote relaxation and to strengthen the body's immune system.

There is little scientific evidence to suggest that this type of therapy has greater benefit than other types of animal assisted therapy. Furthermore, it has been criticized as being extremely costly, not only because of the high price of therapy sessions, but also because of the cost of travel and accommodation for families who must travel to have their child receive the treatment. Parents who consider this therapy should be aware that there are potential risks associated with this therapy, as some dolphins have been known to become aggressive when in captivity.

Training in dolphin assisted therapy

The use of dolphins as an adjunct to therapy is an unregulated practice in both the United States and the United Kingdom. Often, programs are conducted by health care practitioners such as speech, physical, or occupational therapists who are regulated under their profession. Many marine parks or dolphinariums that provide this therapy offer internships, usually lasting for one to two months, for people who are interested in learning the techniques. Some programs, however, are run by people who have no formal training in education or related fields, and who may not fully understand the special needs of children with disabilities.

Recommended resources for dolphin assisted therapy

Literature

Humphries, T.L. (2003) 'Effectiveness of dolphin-assisted therapy as a behavioral intervention for young children with disabilities.' *Bridges, 1*, 6, 1–9.

Marino, L. and Lilienfield, S. (1998) 'Dolphin-assisted therapy: Flawed data, flawed conclusions.' *Anthrozoös, 11*, 4, 194–200.

Nathanson, D.E. (1998) 'Long-term effectiveness of dolphin-assisted therapy for children with severe disabilities.' *Anthrozoös, 11*, 22–32.

Nathanson, D.E., de Castro, D., Friend, H. and McMahon, M. (1997) 'Effectiveness of short-term dolphin-assisted therapy for children with severe disabilities.' *Anthrozoös, 10*, 90–100.

Smith, B. (1996) *Dolphin Assisted Therapy.* Tokyo: Kodansha Publishers.

Smith, B.A. (1983) 'Project Inreach: A program to explore the ability of Atlantic Bottlenose dolphins to elicit communication responses from autistic children.' In A.H. Katcher and A.M. Beck (eds.) *New Perspectives on Our Lives with Companion Animals.* Philadelphia, PA: University of Pennsylvania Press.

Agencies, organizations, and websites

Aquathought Foundation
15921 McGregor Boulevard, Suite 2C
Fort Meyers, FL 33908, USA
Telephone: +1 (941) 437-2958
Website: www.aquathought.com
This organization sponsors the International Dolphin Assisted Therapy and Research Association (IDATRA), which serves to promote the acquisition and dissemination of research in the field of dolphin-assisted therapy.

Dolphin Human Therapy
13605 South Dixie Highway #523
Miami, FL 33176-7252, USA
Telephone: +1 (305) 378-8670
Website: www.dolphinhumantherapy.com

This is the website of David Nathanson, founder of Dolphin Human Therapy. At the time of this writing, Nathanson was attempting to relocate his program due to the problem of hurricanes in South Florida.

Dolphin Reef Eilat
Southern Beach, PO Box 104
Eilat 88100, Israel
Telephone: +972 (8) 6300100
Website: www.dolphinreef.co.il
This center offers dolphin assisted therapy.

Florida's Gulfarium
1010 Miracle Strip Parkway
Fort Walton Beach, FL 32548, USA
Telephone: +1 (850) 243-9096
Website: www.gulfarium.com
This organization sponsors the JF² Dolphin Project, which is a one to two-week program for children with academic, communication, or physical therapy needs. It also provides internships for people interested in DAT.

International Institute of the Dolphin Therapy
97400, Yevpatoriya, Crimea, Kirov Street 49/51
Telephone: +380 (8) 6593-67-41 (Mondays only)
Website: www.dolphintherapy.ru
This program offers dolphin assisted therapy programs in Turkey and Crimea.

Island Dolphin Care
150 Lovelane Place
Key Largo, FL 33037, USA
Telephone: +1 (305) 451-5884
Website: www.islanddolphincare.org
This organization offers a five-day program that combines daily dolphin assisted therapy with classroom therapeutic activities. It also provides training internships.

DORE PROGRAMME

The *DORE programme* is a drug-free treatment for dyslexia and other learning disabilities that was developed by a British businessman, Wynford Dore, whose daughter suffered from severe dyslexia. This treatment was previously referred to as *Dyslexia Dyspraxia Attention Treatment* (*DDAT*). Dore researched the literature for insight as to the neurological problems associated with dyslexia, dyspraxia, and ADHD. He found many references to suggest that these conditions share evidence of poorly developed communication between the *cerebellum* and the *cerebrum* in the brain. Because one of the roles of the cerebellum is to coordinate the nerve processes that contribute to learning, he developed a theory that enhancing maturity of the cerebellum would help learning to become more automatic. The program consists of a series of exercises designed to improve balance and coordination. These are carried out twice per day for approximately ten minutes per session, usually for a period of 12–18 months. The exercise programs are individually prescribed for each child after he or she has taken a series of tests to determine the integrity of various cerebellar functions. Because a certain level of compliance is needed to ensure that the pre and post-assessment measures are accurate, this method is not generally recommended for children under the age of seven years. This program has been widely criticized by the medical community for its high cost and its lack of rigorous scientific study. The few studies that have been published have been criticized for lacking rigor in their design.

Training in the DORE programme

Training is only available to professionals who seek employment in one of the DORE Centers. Two levels of training are provided. A Programme Specialist is responsible for conducting the physiological assessments used to determine the presence of cerebellar problems. These positions are available to persons educated to at least an A level standard with a minimum of one A level in a science subject. Preference is given to candidates with a degree in physiotherapy, psychology, occupational therapy, or another related profession. Programme Specialists are required to attend a five-week training course, and must pass written and clinical examinations. A Programme Practitioner is responsible for initial consultation of prospective patients, interpreting the physiological test results, assessing a patient's suitability for the DORE programme, and monitoring patients' motivation, compliance, and success with the programme. Training for these positions is available to qualified nurses or physiotherapists.

Recommended resources for the DORE programme

Literature

Dore, W. and Brooks, D. (2006) *Dyslexia: The Miracle Cure*. London: Blake Publishing.

Reynolds, D., Nicolson, R.I. and Hambly, H. (2003) 'Evaluation of an exercise-based treatment for children with reading disabilities.' *Dyslexia, 9,* 1, 48–71.

Singleton, C. and Stuart, M. (2003) 'Measurement mischief: A critique of Reynolds, Nicolson & Hambly (2003)' *Dyslexia*, *9*, 3, 151–160.

Snowling, M.J. and Hulme, C. (2003) 'A critique of claims from Reynolds, Nicolson & Hambly (2003) that DDAT is an effective treatment for children with reading difficulties – lies, damned lies and (inappropriate) statistics.' *Dyslexia*, *9*, 2, 127–133.

Agencies, organizations, and websites
DORE Centers
Telephone: +1 (877) 855-3673
Website: www.dorecenters.com
This is the home page for the seven DORE centers located in the United States.
Telephone: +44 (0)870 880 6060
Website: www.dore.co.uk
This is the home page for the twelve DORE centres located in the United Kingdom.

DRAMA THERAPY/PSYCHODRAMA

Drama therapy, also sometimes referred to as *psychodrama*, involves the use of theater and its processes to promote personal growth and mental health. It is used widely in a variety of settings, including hospitals, businesses, mental health centers, and schools. It can involve many different forms of theatrical processes, including simple role-playing activities, group-dynamic games, puppetry, pantomime, and even full-blown theatrical productions with the accompanying props and costumes. For children with developmental disabilities, drama therapy has been proposed as a helpful intervention for facilitating social communication and behaviors, especially for groups of children with Asperger's syndrome or other high functioning autistic disorders. In drama therapy, children have the opportunity to enact relevant events in their lives and to practice reacting to the words and behaviors of other actors in the situation. Some members of the group may serve as the "audience" and act as witnesses to the process of communication and interaction, providing insight as to the success or failure of the process. Drama therapy is not usually used as a stand-alone intervention, but is often incorporated into counseling sessions offered by psychologists, social workers, or other creative arts therapists.

Training in drama therapy/psychodrama

Professionals from a range of disciplines, including psychology, counseling, special education, social work, occupational therapy, art therapy, music therapy, or dance/music therapy may pursue post-graduate training in drama therapy. In the United States, a therapist may become registered as a drama therapist by completing a Master's degree or Doctoral degree in drama therapy from an approved college or university, or by possessing a Master's or Doctoral degree from a related discipline and taking alternative track education requirements, including supervised internship experiences. In the United Kingdom, four universities offer post-graduate training leading to a Master's degree and registration as a dramatherapist.

Recommended resources for drama therapy/psychodrama

Literature

Barnhill, G.P., Cook, K.T., Tebbenkamp, K. and Myles, B.S. (2002) 'The effectiveness of social skills intervention targeting nonverbal communication for adolescents with Asperger Syndrome and related pervasive developmental delays.' *Focus on Autism and Other Developmental Disabilities*, *17*, 112–118.

Blatner, A. (2000) *Foundations of Psychodrama, 4th edn.* New York: Springer Publishing.

Bloom, S., Weber, A.M., Haen, C. and Landy, R. (2004) *Clinical Applications of Drama Therapy in Child and Adolescent Treatment.* New York: Routledge.

Channon, S., Charman, T. and Heap, J. (2001) 'Real-life-type problem-solving in Asperger's Syndrome.' *Journal of Autism and Developmental Disorders*, *31*, 461–469.

Crimmens, P. (2006) *Drama Therapy and Storymaking in Special Education.* London: Jessica Kingsley Publishers.

Agencies, organizations, and websites

British Association of Dramatherapists
Waverly, Battledown Approach
Cheltenham, Gloucestershire GL52 6RE, UK
Telephone: +44 (0)1242 235515
Website: www.badth.org.uk
This is the professional body for dramatherapists in the United Kingdom. It provides information about career training, has a dramatherapist locator, and offers other useful information and links.

National Association for Drama Therapy
15 Post Side Lane
Pittsford, NY 14534, USA
Telephone: +1 (585) 381-5618

Website: www.nadt.org
This is a United States based non-profit organization that promotes
information and advocacy about dramatherapy. It develops criteria for training
and registration of dramatherapists, and sponsors publications and conferences.

EAROBICS®

Earobics® is a commercially produced multimedia approach to literacy learning
that has been successfully implemented in a large number of public schools in
the United States. It has been recognized by the National Institute of Health as
an example of an effective, scientifically-based reading program. As a result, a
number of federal funding sources are available to schools who wish to implement the program into the school's literacy curriculum. It is designed for
students in pre-kindergarten through grade 3, although it may be used for older
students who have significant reading delays.

This program uses entertaining, child-friendly computer games to teach
phonological awareness, listening skills, and phonics skills needed for learning
to read and spell. The program automatically adjusts the level of instruction to
match the individual child's skill level and progress. It also has the capability of
automatically charting the child's progress. Several versions are available, including a version that is suitable for parents to supervise at home. Typically, use of
the program requires the child to spend 15–20 minutes, three times per week,
playing the games.

Training in Earobics®

This is a commercial product that is sold by a number of companies that sell
software for special education needs. Purchase of the software includes instructional material that allows professionals or parents to learn to use the program.
The company that developed the software offers on-site training and support to
schools or other agencies who purchase their product. They also offer family
literacy workshops that are usually held in conjunction with schools that have
decided to purchase the software.

Recommended resources for Earobics®

Literature

Cognitive Concepts, Inc. (1998) *Earobics® Auditory Development and Phonics
    Reading Program.* Evanston, IL: Cognitive Concepts, Inc.

Diehl, S. (1999) 'Listen and learn? A software review of Earobics®. Language,
    speech and hearing services in schools.' *American Speech and Hearing
    Association, 30*, 108–116.

Florida Center for Reading Research (2002) *Earobics® Literacy Launch*.
    www.fcrr.org/FCRRReports/PDF/Earobics_Report.pdf. Accessed 29
    April 2007.

Agencies, organizations, and websites
Earobics® Houghton Mifflin
PO Box 1363
Evanston, IL 60204-1363, USA
Telephone: +1 (888) 328-8199 (USA)
                +1 (847) 328-8099 (outside of the USA)
Website: www.earobics.com
This is the home website for the company that produces Earobics® software. In
addition to offering sales and training support, it provides a comprehensive
overview of the product, information about obtaining funding, including grants
to support the cost of the program in schools, and an overview of relevant
research.

FACILITATED COMMUNICATION

Facilitated communication is a technique used for individuals with severe communication impairments to access communication aids using their hands. This
method was first introduced in the 1970s by an Australian, Rosemary Crossley,
as a method for individuals with severe physical disabilities including cerebral
palsy. It has subsequently been widely used with children who have severe
communication limitations as a result of autism or other developmental disabilities that impair motor planning. The child works with one or more trained
"facilitators" (professionals or non-professionals who have been trained in
the technique) who provide emotional and physical assistance as the person
attempts to communicate through typing, pointing to pictures, or accessing
computer controls. The amount of physical support varies, and may range from
actually holding the person's hand and guiding it towards a picture or key, to providing a light touch reinforcement after the person has made a communicative
effort. As the person gains in communication skill, the amount of facilitation is
gradually reduced to promote independence. Skeptics of the technique argue
that there is limited scientific evidence to support the effectiveness of this intervention. There is also concern that the method may allow facilitators to influence, either knowingly or unknowingly, the thoughts and words expressed by
the disabled individual.

Training in facilitated communication

Facilitated communication is not regulated as a primary intervention, but may be incorporated as one aspect of other educational or communication training. Training in facilitated communication may be included as one aspect of the curriculum for speech-language therapists or special education professionals within the broader context of learning to use various forms of augmentative and alternative communication. University-level courses and workshops are offered through several universities and agencies to introduce the concepts of the technique. Facilitators (professionals and non-professionals) are selected to work with a specific individual, and receive training in the technique as part of that individual's specific treatment plan.

Recommended resources for facilitated communication

Literature

American Academy of Pediatrics Committee on Children with Disabilities (1997) 'Auditory integration therapy and facilitated communication for autism.' *Pediatrics, 102*, 431–433.

Crossley, R. (1994) *Facilitated Communication Training.* New York: Teacher's College Press.

Jacobson, J.W., Mulick, J.A. and Schwartz, A.A. (1995) 'A history of facilitated communication: Science, pseudoscience, and antiscience.' *American Psychologist, 50*, 750–765.

Mostert, M.P. (2001) 'Facilitated communication since 1995: A review of published studies.' *Journal of Autism and Developmental Disabilities, 33,* 2, 219–220.

Agencies, organizations, and websites

CandLE: Communication and Learning Enterprises
48 Station Road
Holywell Green HX4 9AW, UK
Telephone: +44 (0)7904 693302
Website: www.contactcandle.co.uk
This organization is devoted to supporting students with complex communication needs in the United Kingdom.

Deal Communication Centre, Inc.
538 Dandenong Road
Caulfield, Victoria 3162, Australia
Telephone: +61(3) 9509 6324
Website: www.deal.org.au
This is the major center for research, training, and patient services in Australia.

Facilitated Communication Institute

Syracuse University, School of Education, 370 Huntinton Hall

Syracuse, NY 13244-2340, USA

Telephone: +1 (315) 443-9657

Website: http://suedweb.syr.edu/thefci

This is the major center for facilitated communication in the United States, and offers university-level courses as well as workshops and other trainings.

University of Bolton

Deane Road

Bolton BL3 5AB, UK

Telephone: +44 (0)1204 900600

Website: www.bolton.ac.uk

This university offers a BA course in communication therapy, including facilitated communication, along with other forms of augmentative and assistive communication therapies.

FAST FORWORD®

Fast ForWord® is a series of computer-based reading intervention programs that are designed to improve the underlying cognitive skills that students need to improve their English language proficiency and to develop reading skills. The software uses acoustically-altered speech that helps to slow down and enhance the sounds that make up speech so that they can be more easily differentiated. Seven game-like exercises focus on such skills as non-verbal and verbal sound discrimination, vocabulary recognition, and language comprehension. Wearing earphones, students listen to the exercises and respond to demands using a computer mouse. With each successful or unsuccessful click of the mouse, the software adapts to the individual student's skill level, so that the exercises are continually adjusted to challenge and motivate the learner at his or her own level. Training protocols are intensive, ranging from 50 to 100 minutes per day for 4–12 weeks. Separate software allows teachers to track the cognitive gains of students on a daily basis, and provides specific recommendations for instructional intervention to support gains in learning.

Proponents believe that these exercises can strengthen core cognitive and linguistic skills including memory, attention, processing, and sequencing. Research, however, shows mixed results, and purchase of the software programs is costly.

Training in Fast ForWord®

Specific training in Fast ForWord® Language is not required. Scientific Learning, which produces this product, offers free introductory seminars through various professional conferences and meetings. In addition, it offers on-line training seminars about the relationship of brain plasticity to learning.

Recommended resources for Fast ForWord®

Literature

Cohen, W., Hodson, A., O'Hare, A., et al. (2005) 'Effects of computer-based intervention through acoustically modified speech (Fast ForWord®) in severe mixed receptive-expressive language impairment: Outcomes from a randomized controlled trial.' *Journal of Speech, Language and Hearing Research, 48*, 3, 715–729.

Scientific Learning Corporation (2004) 'Improved language skills by children with low reading performance who used Fast ForWord® Language: MAPS for learning.' *MAPS for Learning, 3*, 1, 1–13.

Troia, G.A. (2004) 'Migrant students with limited English proficiency: Can Fast ForWord® make a difference in their language skills and academic achievement?' *Remedial and Special Education, 25*, 6, 353–366.

Valentine, D., Hedrick, M.S. and Swanson, L.A. (2006) 'Effect of an auditory training program on reading, phonemic awareness, and language.' *Perceptual and Motor Skills, 103*, 1, 183–196.

Agencies, organizations, and websites

Neuron Learning

Telephone:+44 (0)207 100 9293 (UK)
            +353 (0)21455 5559 (Republic of Ireland)
Website: www.neuron-learning.co.uk
This website sells Fast ForWord® products and offers learning centres in London, Dublin, and Cork.

Scientific Learning

300 Frank H. Ogawa Plaza, Suite 600
Oakland, CA 94612-2040, USA
Telephone: +1 (888) 665-9707
Website: www.scilearn.com
This company produces and sells the Fast ForWord® software to customers in the United States and Canada.

HOLDING THERAPY

Holding therapy, also referred to as *regulatory bonding therapy*, was developed in the 1970s by Martha G. Welch, a child psychiatrist specializing in problems with parent–child attachment disorders, including autism. It is based upon the assumption that many childhood behavior disorders stem from a stress-related physiological phenomenon in which the parent fails to bond with the child. During holding therapy, an adult (who may or may not be the parent) forcefully restrains the child while talking, poking or tickling to elicit a reaction, and attempting to make eye contact. Even if the child struggles, the adult does not release the child until he or she initiates eye contact with the parent, a sign believed to indicate that the child is ready to interact and bond with the adult. The restraint may last for a few minutes only, or for several hours at a time, and has been criticized for being overly intrusive. Some proponents suggest that the intervention may, in fact, be a type of sensory integrative approach to making contact with the child, since the act of "holding" provides intensive touch and deep pressure stimulation. It has been compared by some to the act of breaking a horse, where the individual eventually acclimates to being touched.

Training in holding therapy

Parents of children with autism or other reactive attachment disorders may contact one of the Martha G. Welch Centers for information about obtaining a personalized consultation or treatment plan. Professional training in the approach is available through one of several Mothering Centers located in New York, Connecticut, and England.

Recommended resources for holding therapy

Literature

Welch, M.G. and Chaput, P. (1988) 'Mother-child holding therapy and autism.' *Pennsylvania Medicine, 91,* 10, 33–38.

Welch, M.G. and Mark, M.E. (1988) *Holding Time: How to Eliminate Conflict, Temper Tantrums, and Sibling Rivalry and Raise Happy, Loving, Successful Children.* New York: Simon & Schuster.

Welch, M.G., Northrup, R.S., Welch-Horan, T.B., Ludwig, R.J., Austin, C.L. and Jacobson, J.S. (2006) 'Outcomes of prolonged parent-child embrace therapy among 102 children with behavioral disorders.' *Complementary Therapy Clinical Practice, 12,* 1, 3–12.

Agencies, organizations, and websites

The Martha G. Welch Center
Website: www.marthawelch.com
This is the official website of the Martha G. Welch Center, and offers descriptions of the approach, research evidence, and an on-line store.

The Mothering Center
952 Fifth Avenue
New York, NY 10021, USA

The Mothering Center
235 Gogenwaugh Road
Cos Cob, CT 06807, USA
Telephone: +1 (206) 661-1413

The Timbergen Trust, The Mothering Center
8 Somerset Road
Teddington, Middlesex TW11 8RS, UK

HYPNOTHERAPY

Hypnotherapy is a set of procedures that teach a child how to self-hypnotize to help control undesired behaviors, habits, or physical symptoms. It is not usually considered an isolated treatment, but may be incorporated into a program of psychotherapeutic intervention provided by a qualified mental health professional. In hypnotherapy, the therapist teaches the child to use relaxation techniques and guided imagery to achieve an altered state of consciousness, sometimes referred to as a *trance*. Once the child is in this altered state, the therapist makes suggestions aimed at producing a change in behavior, anxiety level, or physical symptom. Problems that are commonly addressed through hypnotherapy include anxiety reactions to stress, poor self-esteem, inattention, sleep disturbances, bedwetting, and unpleasant habits such as thumb sucking, hair pulling, or nail biting. Ultimately, the goal is to teach the child to induce self-hypnosis when needed to exercise control over his or herself. People respond to hypnosis in different ways, and some are more open to suggestion than others. Fear of losing control over oneself can inhibit the ability to become hypnotized, but in general, children are more readily hypnotized than adults.

There are many misconceptions about hypnotherapy that must be understood before considering this approach. Many people mistakenly believe that a hypnotist makes a person fall asleep, and then controls that person's mind while they are asleep, leading them to do things they would not otherwise want to do. In fact, hypnosis is a perfectly natural state of mind, one that many children achieve on their own during imaginative play. The child is relaxed, but fully conscious during hypnosis, and cannot be forced to do anything he or she is not willing to do.

Training in hypnotherapy

Many types of professionals, including doctors, psychologists, social workers, and others, use hypnosis as part of their intervention. The techniques are taught through a range of continuing education or certification programs. Hypnotherapy is not formally regulated in either the United States or the United Kingdom, although voluntary certification or registration is offered to professionally licensed medical and mental health professionals through several organizations. It is advisable to avoid consulting with hypnotherapists who are not also licensed as medical or mental health professionals.

Recommended resources for hypnotherapy

Literature

Anbar, R.D. (2006) 'Hypnosis: An important multifaceted therapy.' *Journal of Pediatrics*, *149*, 4, 438–439.

Milling, L.S. and Constantino, C.A. (2000) 'Clinical hypnosis with children: First steps towards empirical support.' *International Journal of Clinical and Experimental Hypnosis*, *48*, 2, 113–137.

Mottin, D.J. (2005) *Raising Your Children with Hypnosis*. Merrimac, NH: National Guild of Hypnotists, Inc.

Olness, K. and Kohen, D.P. (1996) *Hypnosis and Hypnotherapy with Children*. New York: Guilford Press.

Wester, W.C. and Sugarman, L.I. (2002) *Therapeutic Hypnosis with Children and Adolescents*. Bethel, CT: Crown House Publishers.

Agencies, organizations, and websites

American Society of Clinical Hypnosis
140 N. Bloomingdale Road
Bloomingdale, IN 60108, USA
Telephone: +1 (630) 980-4740
Website: www.asch.net
This is an interdisciplinary organization of Master's and doctoral trained practitioners from many professions who practice hypnotherapy. It provides a voluntary certification program available only to professionals who are licensed to provide medical, dental, or psychotherapeutic services. There are number of useful links to other agencies and organizations.

General Hypnotherapy Register
PO Box 204
Lymington SO41 6WP, UK
Telephone: +44 (0)1590 683770
Website: www.general-hypnotherapy-register.com
This agency offers a voluntary registration program for professionals practicing in the United Kingdom, and also offers extensive resource information and links to other sites.

National Council for Hypnotherapy
PO Box 421
Charwelton, Daventry NN11 1AS, UK
Telephone: +44 (0)800 952 0545
Website: www.hypnotherapists.org.uk
This organization offers information, training, and voluntary regulation of hypnotherapy in the United Kingdom. It includes an on-line search service to locate registered hypnotherapists.

National Register of Hypnotherapists and Psychotherapists
Suite B12, Cross Street
Nelson BB9 7EN, UK
Telephone: +44 (0)1282 716839
Website: www.nrhp.co.uk

INTENSIVE INTERACTION

Intensive Interaction refers to a method for supporting and developing non-verbal communication and socialization skills in children and adults with severe or profound learning disabilities, including autism. This approach builds upon the concept of *augmented mothering*, which was proposed by psychologist Geraint Ephraim in 1982. He observed that infants and their parents engage in various types of pre-verbal communication long before the infant learns to speak using words. These interactions involve eye contact, facial expression, non-verbal vocalizations such as cooing or laughing, and hand or body gestures, and are both fun and emotionally rewarding for both the parent and child. Gradually, the parent gains experience in "reading" the infant's behavior and communicative intent, and speaks to the infant using words that apply to the situation. For example, when the infant whines and reaches towards a bottle, the parent might respond by saying "Are you hungry? Do you want your bottle?" and at the same time offers the bottle to the infant. Gradually, the infant develops the ability to communicate more intentionally so that his or her needs are met more easily. In a typically developing child, this eventually leads to understanding what words mean (*receptive vocabulary*) and experimenting with using words to get what he or she wants or needs (*expressive vocabulary*). However, many children or adults with severe or profound learning disabilities including autism are not able to learn language in the same way as a typically developing child. Their tendency to want to avoid social engagement combined with an impaired ability to imitate others can lead to severe communication deficits. Many of the behavioral difficulties observed in these children and adults are believed to relate to their inability to communicate meaningfully with others.

In the 1980s, teachers David Hewett and Melanie Nind built upon Ephraim's theory to develop the model of Intensive Interaction for individuals with profound communication impairment and social withdrawal. They described the importance of understanding that people with autism experience sensation very differently than those without neurological differences. Although every person with autism reacts differently to their sensory world, most are hypersensitive to certain sensory situations, and can become easily stressed or overwhelmed by even small amounts of the offending sensory input. Aggression or acting out behaviors may reflect this sensory distress, and represent an effort to flee from something that is very uncomfortable. Also, many people with autism engage in repetitive, idiosyncratic behaviors that seem non-purposeful to us, but that may serve some meaningful purpose for the person with autism. For example, staring intently at something may help to center the person so that he or she can filter out other stressful stimuli, and touching everything in sight may serve to add information when visual information is distorted and confusing. Hewett and Nind observed that when they imitated the behaviors of people with autism, there was a marked improvement in behavior and social interaction.

Phoebe Caldwell, who resides in Great Britain and is a widely published practitioner of this method, explains that the principle behind Intensive Interaction is to teach parents or other caregivers to carefully observe and think about how the person might experience things differently, and to develop hypotheses about why certain behaviors might exist. They should then calmly respond to the person by using blend of direct imitation and variations of the sounds, behaviors, and body language they have observed. These interactions create emotional engagement. Instead of *directing* the person to perform some specific task, the caregiver allows the person to take the lead role in whatever activities he or she enjoys, joining in and reacting as though the person's preferred activities are mutually enjoyable and of great social importance. Often, the person responds within minutes, recognizing that he or she has found a safe way to communicate with the caregiver. Response to this intervention may include increased eye contact, greater tolerance for physical and social contact with others, a shift from solitary self-stimulation to shared activity, and an increase in non-verbal communicative efforts.

Intensive Interaction was developed in the United Kingdom and is not widely practiced in the United States. Intensive Interaction, the Son-Rise Program® and the DIR®/Floortime model, which are described elsewhere in this book, all share the principle of using imitation of a person's behavior as a way to increase social engagement. The difference is that in Intensive Interaction, imitation has to be interpreted very flexibly as just one of the ways of using a partner's body language.

An advantage to this approach is that is simple, requires no special equipment or props, and is a totally naturalistic intervention that can be employed opportunistically throughout the person's day. Proponents believe that the focus on emotional engagement and stress reduction allows the brain to work more effectively. This may make it easier for the person to respond to more structured interventions that support their ability to learn functional communication and developmental skills.

More research is needed to demonstrate the effectiveness of this approach. The few published studies that do focus on children use small scale or single subject design without controls. Despite this, there is preliminary evidence and considerable anecdotal report suggesting that this intervention helps to increase socially interactive behaviors, and to improve parent satisfaction with their ability to have a meaningful relationship with their child.

Training in Intensive Interaction

This approach may be employed by individuals from a wide range of backgrounds, including parents and other non-professional caregivers. Training is available through reading, workshops, and staff development courses.

Recommended resources for Intensive Interaction

Literature

Caldwell, P. (2007) *From Isolation to Intimacy: Making Friends Without Words.* London: Jessica Kingsley Publishers.

Caldwell, P. (2005) *Finding You Finding Me: Using Intensive Interaction to get in touch with people whose severe learning disabilities are combined with autistic spectrum disorder.* London: Jessica Kingsley Publishers.

Caldwell, P. (2002) *Learning the Language: A Video-Based Resource on Building Relationships with People with Severe Learning Disabilities*. Brighton: Pavilion Publishers.

Ephraim, G. (1982) *Developmental Processes in Mental Handicap: A Generative Structural Approach*. Unpublished Ph.D. Thesis, Brunel University Foundation.

Firth, G. (2006) 'Intensive Interaction: A research review.' *Mental Health and Learning Disabilities Research and Practice, 3*, 1, 53–63.

Heiman, M., Laberg, K.E. and Nordøen (2006) 'Imitative interaction increases social interest and elicited imitation in non-verbal children with autism.' *Infant and Child Development, 15*, 3, 297–309.

Hewett, D. and Nind, M. (1998) *Interaction in Action: Reflections on the Use of Intensive Interaction*. London: David Fulton Publishers.

Kellett, M. (2003) *Implementing Intensive Interaction in Schools: Guidance for Practitioners, Managers, and Co-ordinators*. London: David Fulton Publishers.

Nind, M. and Hewett, D. (2001) *A Practical Guide to Intensive Interaction*. Kidderminster: British Institute of Learning Disabilities Publications.

Nind, M. (2000) 'Teachers' understanding of interactive approaches in special education.' *International Journal of Disability, Development, and Education, 47*, 2: 184–199.

Watson, J. and Fisher, A. (1997) 'Evaluating the effectiveness of Intensive Interaction teaching with pupils with profound and complex learning disabilities.' *The British Journal of Special Education, 24*, 2, 80–87.

Watson, J. and Knight, C. (1991) 'An evaluation of Intensive Interaction teaching with pupils with very severe learning difficulties.' *Child Language Teaching and Therapy, 7*, 3, 310–325.

Zeedyk, S. (2008). *Promoting Social Interaction for Individuals with Communicative Impairments: Making Contact*. London, UK: Jessica Kingsley Publishers.

Agencies, organizations, and websites

David Hewett

Telephone: +44 (0)1920 822027

Email: daveinteract@hotmail.com

Website: www.davehewett.com

David Hewett is one of the founders of the Intensive Interaction approach. His website offers information including publications and courses on the topic. He also provides individual consultation, and welcomes inquiries to discuss questions or ideas about Intensive Interaction.

Intensive Interaction

Website: www.intensiveinteraction.co.uk

This website serves as a resource for people interested in the approach. It offers training events and courses, including training as an advanced practitioner. It also offers publications, DVDs, and links to other relevant organizations.

Leeds Mental Health NHS Trust
Graham Firth, Intensive Interaction Project Coordinator
St. Mary's Hospital, Green Hill Road
Leeds LS12 3QE, UK
Telephone: +44 (0)113 3055160
Website: www.leedsmentalhealth.nhs.uk
Email: graham.firth@leedsmh.nhs.uk
This trust has extensive information and resources pertaining to Intensive Interaction.

Dr. Pete Coia
Clinical Psychology, The Horizon Centre
Fieldhead Hospital, Ouchthorpe Lane
Wakefield WF1 3SP, UK
Dr Pete Coia was also involved in founding the Intensive Interaction approach, about which he writes, speaks at conferences and runs courses at various levels.

Phoebe Caldwell
Email: phoebecaldwell@btopenworld.co.uk/
Phoebe Caldwell runs introductory courses and workshops on Intensive Interaction.

LEARNING BREAKTHROUGH PROGRAM™

The *Learning Breakthrough Program*™ is an activity program that uses balance and sensory activities to develop and refine the basic brain organizations that are believed to form the foundation for learning. It was developed in 1982 by Frank Belgau, who is an educator and director of the Perceptual Motor and Visual Perception Laboratory at the University of Houston, Texas. He proposes that use of the prescribed activities on a structured basis will result in improved vision and coordination, as well as an increased rate of academic achievement.

This program may be incorporated into therapy sessions that are provided by physical therapists, occupational therapists, developmental optometrists, or special educators. It is also, however, promoted as a program that can be provided in the home setting without professional supervision. Parents or professionals who are interested in this program purchase specialized equipment along with activity guides and an interactive DVD. The child watches the DVD that instructs him or her to perform certain activities such as throwing beanbags or performing other challenges to eye-hand coordination while standing on a balance board. Activities should be performed for approximately 20 minutes per day for 8 to 12 months, and are believed to produce permanent changes in brain organization. Although the developers of this program offer many anecdotal reports of learning success using the program, there are no published scientific studies to demonstrate efficacy.

Training in the Learning Breakthrough Program™

This program can be self-taught by reading the program manuals and watching a DVD that is available for sale. In addition, Dr Belgau is available to provide training seminars upon special request.

Recommended resources for the Learning Breakthrough Program™

Literature

No peer reviewed studies were available at the time this book was written.

Agencies, organizations, and websites

Balametrics Incorporated
PO Box 2716
Port Angeles, WA 98362, USA
Telephone: +1 (800) 894-3187
Website: www.balametrics.com
This website offers information about training seminars and also sells program materials.

Learning Breakthrough
10 Sheldrake Lane
Palm Beach Gardens, FL 33418, USA
Telephone: +1 (888) 853-2767
Website: www.learningbreakthrough.com
This is the main site for information about the Learning Breakthrough program, offering information about the theory behind the program, and testimonials about its usefulness. Program materials may also be ordered through this site.

Learning Breakthrough Europe
Website: www.learningbreakthrougheurope.com
This website sells program materials to consumers in the United Kingdom.

LINDAMOOD-BELL®

Lindamood-Bell® refers to a series of supplemental intervention programs designed to help individuals of all ages who struggle with learning the language and concepts needed for learning to read, write, spell, and do math. Each of the programs emphasize the ability to sound out or *decode* the sounds that make up words (also called *phonemes*), to comprehend oral and written language, and to think critically. Each of the programs offer systematic and explicit instruction that is based upon current theory and research regarding the acquisition of reading and critical thinking skills, and have fairly strong research evidence to support the efficacy of the programs. The programs may be of interest to special education teachers, reading specialists, or speech-language therapists. Materials may be purchased for use in individual clinical practice settings, or for classroom use, and can be quite costly. Currently, five programs are offered.

Lindamood Phonemic Sequencing® (LiPS® Program) (formerly called the *ADD Program*, or *Auditory Discrimination in Depth*) stimulates phonemic awareness as students develop awareness of the mouth actions that produce speech sounds. *Visualizing and Verbalizing for Language Comprehension and Thinking® (V/V® Program)* is designed to stimulate the concept imagery that underlies reading comprehension. *Symbol Imagery for Sight Words, Reading, Phonemic Awareness and Spelling® (Seeing Stars® Program)* develops symbol imagery as applied to sight-word development, contextual fluency, spelling, and the speed and stability of phonemic awareness. *On Cloud Nine® Math* develops the ability to image and verbalize the concepts underlying math problems. *Talkies™* is a precursor to the *V/V® Program*, and may be especially helpful in developing the imagery-language connection for children who have significant language delays, such as those with autism.

Intervention is typically intensive, involving several hours per day for 8 to 12 weeks, and can be costly.

Training in Lindamood Bell®

Training in Lindamood-Bell® programs and procedures is available through several types of professional conferences and workshops offered through the Lindamood-Bell Learning Processes, Inc. These programs range in length from one to twelve days, are continually updated to reflect updated theory and practice, and are available to parents as well as professionals. Alternatively, people interested in this approach who cannot attend the training workshops may purchase individual programs that come with a comprehensive teacher's manual, or may purchase videotapes of training sessions.

Recommended resources for Lindamood-Bell®

Literature

Kennedy, K. and Backman, J. (1993) 'Effectiveness of the Lindamood Auditory Discrimination in Depth Program with students with learning disabilities.' *Learning Disabilities Research and Practice, 8*, 4, 253–259.

Pokorni, J., Worthington, C. and Jamison, P. (2004) 'Phonological awareness intervention: Comparison of Fast ForWord, Earobics, and LiPS.' *Journal of Educational Research, 97*, 3, 147–157.

Sadowski, M. and Wilson, V.L. (2006) 'Effects of a theoretically based large-scale reading intervention in a multicultural urban school district.' *American Educational Research Journal, 43*, 1, 137–154.

Torgesen, J., Alexander, A., Wagner, R. *et al.* (2001) 'Intensive remedial instruction for children with severe reading disabilities: Immediate and long-term outcomes from two instructional approaches.' *Journal of Learning Disabilities, 34*, 33–58.

Torgesen, J., Wagner, R., Rashotte, C. *et al.* (1999) 'Preventing reading failure in young children with phonological processing disabilities: Group and individual responses to instruction.' *Journal of Educational Psychology, 91*, 579–593.

Agencies, organizations, and websites

Lindamood-Bell Learning Processes
416 Higuera Street
San Luis Obispo, CA 93401, USA
Telephone: +1 (805) 541-3836
Website: www.lblp.com
This is the home office for the Lindamood-Bell Learning Processes program. It offers information about training throughout the United States and in the United Kingdom, and provides descriptions of the various learning programs.

London Learning Centre
Eardley House, 182–184 Campden Hill Road
London, W8 7AS, UK
Telephone: +44 (0)207 727 0660
Website: www.lblp.co.uk
This is the only approved program offering training and services in the Lindamood-Bell program in the United Kingdom.

MILLER METHOD

The *Miller Method* is a cognitive-developmental systems approach to treating children with autism. It was developed in the 1960s by Arnold Miller, a psychologist, and his wife Eileen Eller-Miller, a speech-language therapist, and is now used in a number of schools in the Northeast United States for children with autism. This method addresses children's body organization, social interaction, and representation issues in both clinical and classroom settings. Its goals are to 1. assess the child's capacity to interact with people and objects, adapt to change, and learn from experience; 2. build the child's awareness of his or her own body as it relates to objects and people; 3. guide children from closed, disconnected, or scattered ways of being into functional, social and communicative exchanges; and 4. provide the necessary transitions from concrete to more abstract symbolic functioning. One premise behind the Miller Method is that children with autism become stalled at early stages of development, and then progress to more advanced stages of development in an incomplete or disordered manner. Because children with autism lack a basic awareness of their body, one of the major interventions in this approach involves having the children balance on various platforms that are elevated approximately 2.5 feet off the floor. The focus involved in maintaining balance and in solving problems such as detouring around obstacles is believed to help the children to learn functional communication and problem solving skills that can then be generalized to situations not involving a raised platform. Another premise is the concept of *systems*, which the Millers define as organized, coherent chunks of behavior that are enacted repetitively. An example of a typical system is the baby who plays peek-a-boo with a parent as he or she learns that something removed from sight is still there and can return to sight. Children have a great deal of investment in maintaining or continuing their systems as a means of progressing through normal developmental stages. Children with autism develop system aberrations that interfere with development. They may become so over involved with something that they cannot detach themselves, as in the child who perseverates in flicking a light switch on and off. Or, they may become so disconnected from objects or people that they lack the motivation to build or sustain relationships with objects or people. Therapy evaluates the individual child's system aberrations, and then uses these to motivate a change in behavior. The Millers also have a unique approach to teaching expressive language, especially useful for non-verbal children with autism. Therapists use sign language combined with words to narrate the child's actions while they are engaged in the activity. This is believed to help the child to relate signs and words to their own actions and develop an inner speech that is critical to developing communication skills. Other specialized interventions are used to help the children to relate to written language using specialized symbols. For example, to teach the written word "cup", the child is shown a picture of a cup, then a stylized picture of a cup made of the letters c-u-p distorted in a way to approximate the shape of a cup, and then finally the written word "cup". This is believed to help the children learn the meaning of printed words that do not visually resemble the object represented by the word.

As a systems approach, this method works best when multiple caregivers are working towards the same goals, using strategies that are incorporated into the child's daily routine. For parents who are able to travel to the Boston area, initial assessment involves approximately two hours, followed by intensive parent training conducted over a three-day period. After the initial period, the intensity of direct therapy varies, but is typically provided for one hour twice weekly. The Millers offer a diagnostic survey that can be completed by parents living too far away to travel to Boston, and offer distance conferencing involving a combination of videotaping, phone conferencing, and internet conferencing. The Millers suggest that their method works best with younger children who are neurologically intact, and when parents are able to provide constant support and a high demand of expectations for the child.

Training in the Miller Method

Professionals from a variety of disciplines may become a Miller Method Specialist by attending a four-day training seminar offered by the Language and Cognitive Development Center, in addition to receiving supervision in managing cases and in successfully passing a written examination. More extended traineeships are available for selected candidates.

Recommended resources for The Miller Method

Literature

Cook, C.O. (1998) 'The Miller Method: A case study illustrating the use of the approach with children with autism in an interdisciplinary setting.' *Journal of Developmental and Learning Disorders, 2*, 2, 231–264.

Miller, A. and Crétien, K. (2007) *The Miller Method: Developing the Capacities of Children on the Autism Spectrum.* London: Jessica Kingsley Publishers.

Miller, A. and Eller-Miller, E. (2000) 'The Miller Method: A cognitive-developmental systems approach for children with body disorganization, social, and communication issues.' In S. Greenspan and S. Weider (eds.) *ICDL Clinical Practices Guidelines: Revising the Standards of Practice for Infants, Toddlers, and Children with Developmental Challenges.* Bethesda, MD: Interdisciplinary Council on Developmental and Learning Disorders.

Agencies, organizations, and websites

The Language and Cognitive Development Center
154 Wells Avenue, Suite 5
Newton, MA 02459, USA
Telephone: +1 (800) 218-5232
Website: www.millermethod.org
This is the official site for the Miller Method. It offers evaluation and treatment
in the method, as well as a variety of other resources for children with autism.

MULTISENSORY READING INSTRUCTION

There are many different approaches to teaching language and literacy skills to
children with reading disorders that occur as a result of developmental disabilities. Many of these focus on multisensory instructional practices that are
believed to promote non-language mental representations of words, and are
based upon principles first promoted in the 1930s by Samuel T. Orton, a
neuropsychiatrist and pathologist, and Anna Gillingham, a psychologist and
educator. Together, they introduced the *Orton-Gillingham Approach* to reading
instruction, which is an intensive, sequential, phonics-based program of
instruction that incorporates visual, auditory, tactile and *kinesthetic* (sense of
feeling through touch and movement) pathways for learning. Numerous other
reading programs have subsequently been introduced that are based on the principles of Orton-Gillingham, the most popular of which include the *Wilson
Reading System* and the *Specialized Program for Individualizing Reading Excellence
(SPIRE)*. Although the specific methods of each program differ slightly, the
basic content and principles of instruction are similar. They provide systematic
instruction in the five important aspects of reading: *phonemic awareness* (knowledge of the letter sounds), *phonics* (connecting sounds with letters or groups of
letters in words), *reading fluency* (the ability to read text rapidly and correctly),
vocabulary, and comprehension. Instruction is intensive, occurs individually or
in small groups, and is diagnostic and prescriptive in nature, requiring the
program to be individualized to meet the needs of each child. Teaching involves
all learning pathways, sometimes referred to as *VAKT* (for visual-auditory-
tactile-kinesthetic), although the exact method varies, and may include tactile
tracing of letters or tapping out sounds with the fingers as words are *decoded*
(sounded out).

There is abundant evidence to support the effectiveness of these programs
with children who have significant reading disabilities. In fact, there is growing
evidence that the brain systems responsible for reading can actually change and
improve over time, given effective reading instruction. However, the intensity

of some of these interventions makes it difficult to implement them effectively in some school settings.

Training in multisensory reading instruction

Most undergraduate and graduate students in special education or literacy education programs are exposed to multisensory teaching strategies. However, knowledge and experience with the programs that are available varies widely, and consumers are cautioned to be sure that a teacher has had specific training in the method used. The Academy of Orton-Gillingham Practitioners and Educators offers a lengthy process to become certified in their approach, and offers four levels of membership based on the level of training and supervision of the member. Training in the other multisensory reading approaches is usually available through the publisher of the program materials, or through other professional continuing education programs.

Recommended resources for multisensory reading instruction

Literature

Birsh, J.R. (2005) *Multisensory Teaching of Basic Language Skills.* Baltimore, MD: Paul H. Brookes Publishing Co.

Gillingham, A. and Stillman, B.W. (1997) *The Gillingham Manual: Remedial Training for Students with Specific Disability in Reading, Spelling, and Penmanship, 8th edn.* Cambridge, MA: Educators Publishing Service.

Henry, M.K. and Brickley, S.G. (eds.) (1999) *Dyslexia: Samuel T. Orton and his Legacy.* Baltimore, MD: The International Dyslexia Association.

National Reading Panel (2000) *Teaching Children to Read: An Evidence-Based Assessment of the Scientific Research Literature on Reading and its Implications for Reading Instruction (NIH Publication 00-4754).* Washington, DC: National Institute of Child Health and Human Development.

Oakland, T., Black, J.L., Stanford, G., Nussbaum, N.L. and Balise, R.R. (1998) 'An evaluation of the dyslexia training program: A multisensory method for promoting reading in students with reading disabilities.' *Journal of Learning Disabilities, 31,* 2, 140–147.

O'Connor, J.R. and Wilson, B.A. (1995) 'Effectiveness of the Wilson Reading System used in public school training.' In McIntyre, C. and Pickering, J. (eds.) *Clinical Studies of Multisensory Structured Language Education.* Salem, OR: International Multisensory Structured Language Education Council.

Ritchey, K.D. and Goeke, J.L. (2006) 'Orton-Gillingham and Orton-Gillingham- based reading instruction: A review of the literature.' *The Journal of Special Education, 40,* 3, 171–183.

Shaywitz, S. (2003) *Overcoming Dyslexia: The New and Complete Science-Based Program for Reading Problems at Any Level.* New York: Alfred A. Knopf.

Shaywitz, S.E. and Shaywitz, B.A. (2005) 'Dyslexia (specific reading disability).' *Biological Psychiatry, 57*, 11, 1301–1309.

Agencies, organizations, and websites

Academy of Orton-Gillingham Practitioners and Educators
PO Box 234
Amenuia, NY 12501-0234, USA
Telephone: +1 (845) 373-8919
Website: www.ortonacademy.org
This organization offers information about the Orton-Gillingham approach for the treatment of dyslexia, as well as information about training and certification programs sponsored by the academy. It also offers a listing of educators certified in the Orton-Gillingham approach.

International Dyslexia Association
40 York Road, 4th Floor
Baltimore, MD 21204-5202, USA
Telephone: +1 (410) 296-0232
Website: www.interdys.org
This organization, formerly called the Orton Dyslexia Society, promotes literacy through research, education, and advocacy, with a focus on methods based on the Orton-Gillingham approaches.

International Reading Association
PO Box 8139, 800 Barksdale Road
Newark, DE 19714-8139, USA
Telephone: +1 (800) 336-7323
Website: www.reading.org
This is a member organization that serves to promote professional development, research, practice, and policy that improves the quality of reading instruction. It offers a range of resources, products, and continuing education opportunities.

Institute for Multi-Sensory Education (IMSE)
1000 S. Old Woodward, Suite 105
Birmingham, MI 48009, USA
Telephone: +1 (800) 646-9788
Website: www.orton-gillingham.com
This is a national teacher training organization specializing in Orton-Gillingham instruction. It offers a wide array of training and product resources.

The Florida Center for Reading Research
City Centre Building, 227 N. Bronough Street, Suite 7250
Tallahassee, FL 32301, USA
Telephone: +1 (850) 644-9352
Website: www.fcrr.org
This organization offers a range of resources pertaining to best practices in reading instruction, including a database of comprehensive summaries of various reading programs and methods.

Wilson Academy
Website: www.wilsonacademy.com
This is an on-line resource designed to provide professional development courses, references, and instructional materials related to the Wilson Reading System.

MUSIC THERAPY

Music therapy is an allied health profession that uses music as a tool within the context of a therapeutic relationship to address the physical, psychological, cognitive, and motoric needs of individuals. Music is thought to be an effective therapeutic medium because it is non-verbal, non-threatening, and naturally motivating to most people. After assessing the individual needs of the child, music therapists create a treatment plan that may involve having the child create music, sing, listen to, or move in response to music. Musical talent is not required, although many children with autism have unusual sensitivities to music and may respond to the therapy especially well. Simple musical games like passing an object back and forth to a tune may help the child to develop eye contact. Songs that use lyrics composed like social stories can be used to practice social skills. Simple vocal music activities may be helpful for children who have difficulty learning to communicate verbally. Music can help the autistic child to learn the rhythm, stress, flow, and inflection of speech, and can help to break the patterns of monotonous speech common among these children. Music therapy can be provided through individual sessions, but is more frequently offered through group activities in institutional or educational settings.

Training in music therapy

In both the United States and the United Kingdom, music therapists are graduates of an approved baccalaureate program in music therapy that includes coursework in music and music therapy, psychology, as well as biological, social and behavioral sciences, and the study of disabling conditions. Following completion of studies and a supervised internship, students are eligible for admission to a certification examination. In the United States, therapists who have successfully completed this examination use the initials MT-BC following their name.

Recommended resources for music therapy

Literature

Alvin, J. and Warwick, A. (1992) *Music Therapy for the Autistic Child, 2nd edn*. New York: Oxford University Press.

Lorenzato, K.I. and Roskam, K. (2005) *Filling a Need While Making Some Music: A Music Therapist's Guide to Pediatrics*. London: Jessica Kingsley Publishers.

Robb, S.L. (ed.) (2003) *Music Therapy in Pediatric Healthcare: Research and Evidence-Based Practice*. Silver Spring, MD: American Music Therapy Association.

Walworth, D. (2007) 'The use of music therapy within the SCERTS Model for children with autism spectrum disorder.' *Journal of Music Therapy, 44*, 1, 2–22.

Wigram, T. and Gold, C. (2006) 'Music therapy in the assessment and treatment of autism spectrum disorder: Clinical application and research evidence.' *Child Care and Health Development, 32*, 5, 535–542.

Agencies, organizations, and websites

American Music Therapy Association, Inc.
8455 Colesville Road, Suite 1000
Silver Spring, MD 20910, USA
Telephone: +1 (301) 589-3300
Website: www.musictherapy.org
This is the professional organization for music therapists in the United States, featuring a range of products and resources.

Certification Board for Music Therapists
506 E. Lancaster Avenue, Suite 102
Downingtown, PA 19335, USA
Telephone: +1 (800) 765-2268
Website: www.cbmt.org
This organization offers accreditation for schools offering training in music therapy, and serves as the national certification board for music therapists in the United States.

Music Therapy Charity
2 Charles Street
London W1X 4HA, UK
Website: www.musictherapy.org.uk

The Association of Professional Music Therapists
61 Church Hill Road
East Barnet, Hertfordshire EN4 8SY, UK
Telephone: +44 (0)208 440 4153
Website: www.apmt.org
This is the professional organization in the United Kingdom that is responsible
for regulating the practice of music therapy.

NEUROFEEDBACK

Neurofeedback is a specialized type of biofeedback that is used for children with a
variety of learning and behavioral differences. Depending on the provider, it
may also be referred to as *neurotherapy, neurobiofeedback,* or *EEG biofeedback.* The
most common and well documented use of neurofeedback has been with
children diagnosed with ADHD. The intervention involves placing electrodes
on the child's unshaven head to measure brainwave activity as recorded on an
electroencephalogram (EEG). The EEG provides a map of the child's mental
function by comparing five different brainwaves. *Beta waves* are the fastest waves
and are present when a person is attentive. For children with ADHD, the goal is
to increase their beta waves. *SMR waves* are a subcategory of beta waves, and
occur when a person is quietly focused to prepare for a physical challenge. *Alpha
waves* are slower waves and are the brainwaves of relaxation; children with high
levels of stress or anxiety are taught to increase their alpha waves. *Theta waves* are
very slow and are the predominant pattern when a person is daydreaming or
almost falling asleep. *Delta waves* are the slowest waves and are most present
during deep sleep. When the child is connected to the EEG, he or she is exposed
to a video display, sounds, or vibration, and is then taught to develop voluntary
control of brainwave activity. As brainwave activity changes, the therapist either
positively rewards the child, or provides negative feedback, thus gradually
shaping the child's conscious control over brain activity. Proponents believe that
any changes in control over brainwave activity will be permanent.

Neurofeedback can be costly, as it requires many sessions and is often not
covered by insurance. Also, the child must be actively engaged in the program,
meaning that he or she must be old enough to comply with the procedures and
to want to make positive changes. Older children and adults may show less
improvement than younger children, however, because their brains have
matured and are more resistant to change.

Training in neurofeedback

Neurofeedback is often incorporated into the practice of psychologists and psychotherapists, who must be licensed by their regulatory agencies. The practice of neurofeedback does not require specific training. Most therapists interested in the intervention attend various seminars or continuing education courses. They may or may not have formal training in physiology or computer technology. Certification in biofeedback (including neurofeedback) is available, but is not required for practice.

Recommended resources for neurofeedback

Literature

Demos, J.N. (2004) *Getting Started with Neurofeedback*. New York: W.W. Norton & Co.

Evans, J.R. and Abarbnanel, A. (1999) *An Introduction to Quantitative EEG and Neurofeedback*. San Diego, CA: Academic Press.

Foks, M. (2005) 'Neurofeedback training as an educational intervention in a school setting: How the regulation of arousal states can lead to improved attention and behavior in children with special needs.' *Educational and Child Psychology, 22*, 3, 67–77.

Gruzelier, J. and Egner, T. (2005) 'Critical validation studies of neurofeedback.' *Child and Adolescent Psychiatric Clinics of North America, 14*, 1, 83–104.

Gruzelier, J., Egner, T. and Vernon, D. (2006) 'Validating the efficacy of neurofeedback for optimising performance.' *Progress in Brain Research, 159*, 421–431.

Heinrich, H., Gevensleben, H. and Strehl, U. (2007) 'Annotation: Neurofeedback-train your brain to train behaviour.' *Journal of Child Psychology and Psychiatry and Allied Disciplines, 48*, 1, 3–16.

Larsen, S. (2006) *The Healing Power of Neurofeedback*. Rochester, VT: Healing Arts Press.

Monastra, V.J. (2005) 'Electroencephalographic biofeedback (neurotherapy) as a treatment for attention deficit disorder: Rationale and empirical foundation.' *Child and Adolescent Psychiatric Clinics of North America, 14*, 1, 53–82.

Scolnick, B. (2005) 'Effects of electroencephalographic biofeedback with Asperger's syndrome.' *International Journal of Rehabilitation Research, 28*, 2, 159–163.

Agencies, organizations, and websites

Biofeedback Certification Institute of America

10200 W 44th Avenue, Suite 310

Wheat Ridge, CO 80033-2840, USA

Telephone: +1 (303) 420-2902

Website: www.bcia.org

This organization was created to establish and maintain professional standards for the provision of biofeedback services, and to certify those who meet these standards.

Biofeedback Foundation of Europe

PO Box 555

3800 AN Amersfoort, The Netherlands

Telephone: +31 (0) 84 83 84 696

Website: www.bfe.org

This organization promotes a greater awareness of neurofeedback among the world's health professionals through training and research activities.

EEG Info

22020 Clarendon Street, Suite 305

Woodland Hills, CA 91367, USA

Telephone: +1 (818) 373-1334

Website: www.eeginfo.com

This site offers extensive information about neurofeedback, including training for professionals, and links to international providers.

EEG Neurofeedback

PO Box 895

St Albans AL1 9EH, UK

Telephone: +44 (0)1727 874292

Website: www.eegneurofeedback.com

This is a comprehensive provider of neurofeedback training and services in the United Kingdom.

International Society for Neurofeedback and Research

1925 Francisco Boulevard E. #12

San Rafael, CA 94901, USA

Telephone: +1 (415) 485-1344

Website: www.isnr.org

This organization offers extensive information about neurofeedback including references organized by topic and a listing of international members.

Society of Applied Neuroscience

Telephone: Dr Edwin Verstraeten, Secretary, +44 (0)1792 295908 (UK)

Website: www.applied-neuroscience.org

This is the society to which most European practitioners of neurofeedback belong.

PICTURE EXCHANGE COMMUNICATION SYSTEM (PECS)

The *Picture Exchange Communication System (PECS)*, pronounced *pex*, is a specialized augmentative/alternative communication system designed to teach children and adults with severe communication deficits, such as autism, to learn how to initiate communication. It was developed in 1985 by Andy Bondy, a clinical psychologist, and Lori Frost, a speech-language therapist, as part of a comprehensive educational program that incorporates elements of applied behavior analysis, called the *Pyramid Approach to Education*. The logic behind this program is that most individuals with autism prefer to learn through visual media, so the use of pictures to teach communication makes sense. Key to the program is identifying what types of reinforcers will be particularly motivating to the individual child, and then creating a picture card of the items. Communication skills are then taught through six phases of learning. Initially, children are taught to exchange a simple picture of a highly desired item (such as a special toy or a piece of candy) with an adult who immediately responds to the request. Gradually, the adult moves farther away and moves the pictures out of reach so the child has to seek out both the picture and the adult to obtain the desired item. This teaches the child to be persistent in communicative efforts. Once this is learned, the child is taught to discriminate between more discrete pictures of desired items. For example, if the child has a particular taste for a type of candy, he or she may be presented with pictures of several similar types of candy, and must select the correct picture before receiving reinforcement. Later stages of training teach the child to put pictures together to form sentence strips, to ask questions using picture symbols, and to make comments about things they encounter in their environment. In the initial phase of training, an adult works closely with the child in a highly structured setting, such as a therapy session. However, as the child gains mastery, the pictures are incorporated into all aspects of the child's day, requiring carry-over by all professionals and family members who have contact with the child. Although PECS is designed to teach children to communicate non-verbally through these picture symbols, some children will also begin to use verbal language as a result of this training.

PECS is widely used by teachers, speech therapists, and others who work with children with autism. However, the developers of the program caution that using pictures alone does not constitute a PECS program, and that providers of this intervention must be trained in the approach. There is good research evidence to support the effectiveness of this intervention in teaching non-verbal communication skills. Its effectiveness in teaching spoken language is more equivocal.

Training in PECS

Pyramid Educational Consultants, Inc. is the only approved provider of training and consultation in PECS and the Pyramid Approach to Education. A number of training workshops are offered worldwide. PECS Implementer certification involves attendance at a two-day workshop plus ongoing consultation from Pyramid Educational Consultants, and is the minimal level of training required to use the PECS program. More advanced workshops are available to individuals or teams who wish to integrate PECS programs into schools or other programs, or for those who wish to supervise others in the use of PECS.

Recommended resources for PECS

Literature

Carr, D. and Felce, J. (2007) 'Brief report: Increase in production of spoken words in some children with autism after PECS teaching to phase III.' *Journal of Autism and Developmental Disorders, 37*, 4, 780–787.

Charlop-Christy, M., Carpenter, M., Le, L., Leblanc, L. and Keller, K. (2002) 'Using the Picture Exchange Communication System (PECS) with children with autism: Assessment of PECS acquisition, speech, social-communicative behavior, and problem behavior.' *Journal of Applied Behavior Analysis, 35*, 213–231.

Frost, L. and Bondy, A. (2002) *PECS: The Picture Exchange Communication System, 2nd edn.* Newark, DE: Pyramid Educational Consultants, Inc.

Howlin, P., Gordon, R.K., Pasco, G., Wade, A. and Charman, T. (2007) 'The effectiveness of Picture Exchange Communication System (PECS) training for teachers of children with autism: A pragmatic, group randomised controlled trial.' *Journal of Child Psychology and Psychiatry, 48*, 5, 473–481.

Tincani, M. (2004) 'Comparing the Picture Exchange Communication System and sign language training for children with autism.' *Focus on Autism and Other Developmental Disabilities, 19,* 152–163.

Web, T., Baker, S. and Bondy, A. (2005) 'Picture Exchange System.' In L. Wankoff (ed.) *Innovative Methods in Language Intervention* (pp. 111–139). Austin, TX: Pro-Ed Inc.

Agencies, organizations, and websites

Pyramid Educational Consultants, Inc.

13 Garfield Way

Newark, DE 19713, USA

Telephone: +1 (888) 732-7462

Website: www.pecs.com

This is the company that sponsors training in PECS and the Pyramid Approach to education. It offers an overview of the program, information about training opportunities, products, extensive citings of research using PECS, links to international PECS sites, and links to other sites relating to autism.

Pyramid Educational Consultants UK, Ltd.

Pavillion House, 6 Old Steine

Brighton BN1 1EJ, UK

Telephone: +44 (0)1273 609555

Website: www.pecs.org.uk

PLAY ATTENTION®

Play Attention® is a computer-based program that was introduced in 1996 as an intervention to improve attention and cognitive skills in children and adults with ADHD and other problems affecting attentional focus. It uses technology that was originally developed by the National Aeronautics and Space Administration (NASA) to help pilots stay awake and focused, and to reduce errors resulting from pilot inattention. The program utilizes a bike helmet that is lined with sensors that measure brainwaves. The student wears the helmet while looking at a computer screen and using mind control to play a series of games and exercises. The computer produces visual feedback that helps the user to control his or her level of concentration. Once the student has mastered the software, concentration is generalized to real life situations by wearing the helmet during homework. In this application, the software signals the student if he or she is insufficiently attending to the homework assignment. The program also offers guidance on using behavioral reinforcement strategies to help the student to transfer new skills to the classroom, such as learning to read attentively or to pay attention to the teacher during lessons. Unlike biofeedback or neurofeedback, the developers of this program make no claims that the program alters brain function in any way. Instead, they claim that use of the program produces cognitive changes that help the user to become more aware of his or her level of concentration at any time.

This program is recommended for students age six through adult, although it may be used for younger students. It is recommended that training occur twice weekly for 30 to 40 minutes per session. Proponents suggest that 40 to 60 hours of training are needed to achieve permanent results. Evidence for the effectiveness of this intervention is limited to a few case studies and anecdotal reports of success.

Training in Play Attention®

As a commercial product, purchase of the Play Attention® system includes all materials and training instructions. Once registered as a user, the company offers free technical support and mentoring assistance. For a fee, professionals may become certified as a Play Attention® Provider which allows access to training around marketing strategies for the program.

Recommended resources for Play Attention®

Literature

Ashton, T. (n.d.) *Improving attention, reducing behavior problems, and bolstering self-esteem: The many benefits of Play Attention.* Available at http://jset.unlv.edu/16.2/asseds/ashton.html, accessed 25 June 2007.

Siglin, J.A. (2000) 'Play Attention®: Focusing on success.' *Intervention in School and Clinic, 36*, 2, 122–124.

Agencies, organizations, and websites

Unique Logic and Technology
1 Botany Drive
Asheville, NC 28805, USA
Telephone: +1 (800) 788-6786 (USA)
+1 (828) 225 5522 (outside of the USA)
Website: www.playattention.com
This is the website of the company that produces and sells the Play Attention® technology. It offers free demonstrations and a range of information about the technology suitable for parents and professionals.

PRIMARY MOVEMENT® PROGRAM

Primary Movement® is a unique movement program that is based on the premise that some children with dyslexia or other learning differences have failed to proceed through normal stages of motor development, and that this contributes to problems with learning to read. All children are born with certain primitive movement patterns (*reflexes*) that emerge during the fetal stage and are important for the young infant's survival. Each primitive reflex serves a particular function for the child, but is no longer needed after a certain length of time as the child matures. Once a reflex has outlived its purpose, it becomes integrated into the central nervous system, and is no longer observed, although it remains dormant within the central nervous system. Some of these primitive reflexes are well known. For example, all young infants have a *rooting reflex* which helps them to locate the mother's nipple for feeding. When one cheek is gently stroked, the infant will turn his or her head in that direction so that the head is in a better position for suckling. Other primitive reflexes are less well known. For example, the *asymmetric tonic neck reflex (ATNR)* is present at birth. When the infant is lying on his or her back and the head is turned to one side, the limbs respond in a predictable manner. The arm that is closest to the face will extend in order to provide some protection for the face, and the other arm bends to protect the back of the head. This reflex is no longer needed when the infant has gained sufficient voluntary control over body movements to protect him or herself through more purposeful efforts.

Proponents of the Primary Movement® Program have observed that in some children with dyslexia or other learning problems, certain primitive reflexes persist long after they should have become integrated into the central nervous system. They believe that practice and repetition of the primitive reflex patterns actually help them to more easily integrate. Teachers or other professionals who are trained in the program observe the child to determine which reflexes need to be integrated, and then design an activity program that involves practice and repetition of the necessary reflex patterns. The activities are very child friendly, using interesting songs and rhythmic movements, and are practiced for 10–15 minutes per day, five days per week. Some schools use the movement activities as a natural way to transition from one learning activity to another, while others integrate the exercises into the school's physical education curriculum. Once the activities have been selected, they can also be easily carried out at home. To date, limited research has been conducted to evaluate the potential success of this program in improving cognitive or academic performance.

Training in the Primary Movement® Program

Training in the Primary Movement® Program is available in the United Kingdom, Ireland, and Australia. Stage 1 training is a three-day course open to teachers and other professionals interested in this approach for children ages four through seven. Stage 2 training is available to those who have completed Stage 1 training, and provides instruction for working with older children and adults.

Recommended resources for the Primary Movement® Program

Literature

Jordon-Black, J.A. (2005) 'The effects of the Primary Movement® programme on the academic performance of children attending ordinary primary school.' *Journal of Research in Special Education Needs*, 5, 3, 101–111.

McPhillips, M. and Sheehy, N. (2004) 'Prevalence of persistent primary reflexes and motor problems in children with reading difficulties.' *Dyslexia*, *10*, 4, 316–338.

Agencies, organizations, and websites

Primary Movement®

The Foyer, 3–5 Malone Road

Belfast BT9 6RT, Northern Ireland

Telephone: +44 (0)2890 222182 (UK)

+353 (0)4890 222182 (Republic of Ireland)

+44 (0)2890 222182 (all other countries)

Website: www.primarymovement.org

RHYTHMIC ENTRAINMENT INTERVENTION (REI THERAPY)

Entrainment is a natural phenomenon that causes two or more vibrating bodies to become synchronized in their rhythm. This has been documented in many areas of human function. For example, respiration and heart rates can be modified through auditory input, and subtle body movements of people can synchronize during normal conversation. *Rhythmic entrainment intervention (REI)* is a music-medicine program that is based on the principle of entrainment, and is used primarily for children with developmental and learning problems, such as autism spectrum disorders and ADHD. The specific intervention was derived from two healing techniques, *shamanic drumming* and *rhythm healing*, which have been used for thousands of years to treat various physical and psychological problems. Following an assessment of the child's unique cognitive and behavioral characteristics, the REI provider develops two personalized CD percussion recordings, with rhythms selected to address specific areas of concern, such as communication skills, attention span, self-stimulatory behavior, aggression, or anxiety. Through the process of entrainment, the auditory rhythms chosen for the child are believed to stimulate the central nervous system and ultimately to improve brain function. The recording is played once per day for a period of eight to twelve weeks, and proponents believe that the effects can be long lasting. REI therapy has not been subjected to rigorous scientific review, and is therefore considered an unproven intervention.

Training in rhythmic entrainment intervention

This intervention is not regulated in the United States or the United Kingdom. Health care professionals may become authorized providers of REI by attending a one day seminar.

Recommended resources for rhythmic entrainment intervention

Literature

Clayton, M., Sager, R. and Will, U. (2003) *In Time with the Music: The Concept of Entrainment and its Significance for Ethnomusicology.* Available at www.ccs.fau.edu/~large/Publications/ClaytonSagerWill2004.pdf, accessed 14 January 2007.

Maxfield, M. (1990) *Effects of Rhythmic Drumming on EEG and Subjective Experience* (Doctoral Dissertation). San Francisco Institute of Transpersonal Psychology.

Strong, J. (2004) *Rhythmic Entrainment Intervention (Rei): Blending Ancient Techniques with Modern Research Findings.* Available at www.reiinstitute.com/openear2004.html, accessed 29 June 2007.

Strong, J. (1998) *Rhythmic Entrainment Intervention: a Theoretical Perspective.* Available at www.reiinstitute.com/rei-article.html, accessed 29 June 2007.

Agencies, organizations, and websites

REI Institute
55 Lime Kiln Road
Lamy, NM 87540, USA
Telephone: +1 (800) 659-6644
Website: www.reiinstitute.com
This organization offers training centers, personalized REI programs, and pre-recorded generalized CDs.

SENSORY INTEGRATION THERAPY

Sensory integration therapy (SI) is based on theoretical assumptions that were first introduced by Jean Ayres, who was trained both as an occupational therapist and a psychologist, in the early 1970s. Dr Ayres defined sensory integration as a normal developmental process involving the ability of the child's central nervous system to organize sensations from the environment and from within the body to make adaptive responses necessary for learning and for behavioral regulation. Of special interest are sensory processing related to the *vestibular system* (which involves gravity, motion, balance, and eye-hand coordination), the *proprioceptive system* (involved with body awareness and sub-conscious control of movement), and the tactile system. Signs of sensory processing difficulties may include over- or under-sensitivity to certain sensory experiences, abnormally high or low activity level, poorly organized behavior, poor coordination and motor learning, or delays in language development or academic progress despite adequate intelligence. Sensory integration therapy is most commonly used within occupational therapy programs, and is one aspect of a more generalized focus on the child's occupational functioning, although some of the techniques may be used by teachers or other professionals. It is one of the most common approaches used by occupational therapists who treat children with autism, attention deficit disorders, or other learning disabilities. Therapy programs incorporating sensory integration principles commonly involve one or two sessions per week for a period of at least six months, although the recommended frequency and duration will vary from child to child. After evaluating how the child responds to different sensory inputs, different motoric challenges, and different aspects of social interaction, the therapist designs a program that encourages the child to engage in playful activities that demand challenging adaptive responses. An important part of the therapy is understanding the profound influence that different types of sensory input have on a child's behavior and learning, then modifying the sensory environment so that the child gets exactly what he or she needs in order to learn. This is sometimes referred to as designing a *sensory diet* for the child. A sensory diet may incorporate environmental modifications, such as reducing unnecessary distractions, changing lighting, or modifying classroom tools and materials. It may also involve specific sensory stimulation techniques, such as wearing a weighted vest to promote calming, or providing small toys to hold and fidget with to promote attention. Teaching parents and other caregivers how to carry over strategies into everyday situations is considered an important element of the therapy program.

Training in sensory integration therapy

Sensory integration therapy is most commonly provided by occupational therapists, and all occupational therapists are introduced to the theory as part of their basic professional education. Certification in one assessment battery, the Sensory Integration and Praxis Tests (SIPT) is available to therapists, and most therapists who have achieved this certification have undergone other types of continuing education as well. However, the SIPT is not an appropriate test for all children and many experienced therapists use alternative methods to identify S1 dysfunction. Parents should be aware that certification in the SIPT does not attest to the therapist's skill and experience in providing treatment, but only attests to having had training in administering the SIPT test battery. Competency is gained through a combination of continuing education, mentoring, and clinical experience. When selecting a therapist, look for someone who has certification plus other continuing education in the approach, and who has received supervision in clinical practice with children who have similar problems.

Recommended resources for sensory integration therapy

Literature

Ayres, A.J. (1979) *Sensory Integration and the Child*. Los Angeles, CA: Western Psychological Services.

Bundy, A.C., Lane, S., Murray, E.A. and Fisher, A.G. (2002) *Sensory Integration: Theory and Practice, 2nd edn*. Philadelphia: F.A. Davis.

Cohn, E.S. (2001) 'Parent perspectives of occupational therapy using a sensory integration approach.' *American Journal of Occupational Therapy, 55,* 285–294.

Horowitz, L.J. and Rost, C. (2007) *Helping Hyperactive Kids—A Sensory Integration Approach: Techniques and Tips for Parents and Professionals*. Alameda, CA: Hunter House Publishers.

Kranowitz, C.S. (1998) *The Out-of-Sync Child: Recognizing and Coping with Sensory Integration Dysfunction*. New York: Berkeley Publishing Group.

Miller, L.J., Coll, J.R. and Schoen, S.A. (2007) 'A randomized controlled pilot study of the effectiveness of occupational therapy for children with sensory modulation disorder.' *American Journal of Occupational Therapy, 61,* 2, 228–238.

Schaaf, R.C. and Miller, L.J. (2005) 'Occupational therapy using a sensory integrative approach for children with developmental disabilities.' *Mental Retardation Research Reviews, 11,* 2, 143–148.

Smith, S.A., Press, B., Koenig, K.P. and Kinnealey, M. (2005) 'Effects of sensory integration intervention on self-stimulating and self-injurious behavior.' *American Journal of Occupational Therapy, 59,* 4, 418–425.

Agencies, organizations, and websites

American Occupational Therapy Association, Inc.
PO Box 31220
Bethesda, MD 20824-1220, USA
Telephone: +1 (301) 652-2682
              +1 (800) 377-8555 (TDD)

Website: www.aota.org
This is the official organization of occupational therapists in the United States.

British Association of Occupational Therapists
106–114 Borough High Street
London SE1 1LB, UK
Telephone: +44 (0)207 357 6480
Website: www.cot.org.uk
This is the official organization of occupational therapists in the United
Kingdom.

Sensory Integration International
PO Box 5339
Torrance, CA 90510-5339, USA
Telephone: +1 (310) 787-8805
This organization offers certification in the Sensory Integration and Praxis tests,
and provides a registry of certified therapists.

American Occupational Therapy Foundation
Website: www.aotf.org
This organization offers a thorough review of sensory integration research.

Western Psychological Services
12031 Wilshire Boulevard
Los Angeles, CA 90025-1251, USA
Telephone: +1 (800) 648-8857
Website: www.wpspublish.com
This company offers certification in the Sensory Integration and Praxis Tests in
affiliation with the University of Southern California, and provides a registry of
certified therapists.

SIGN LANGUAGE

Learning to communicate is a major issue for most children with autism
spectrum disorders. As many as half of children with autism do not talk at all,
while others may have rich vocabularies, but struggle with the use of language in
the context of socially appropriate communication. The inability to communicate basic wants and needs can be a significant source of frustration for the child
with autism, and may be a contributing factor to the tantrums, self-injurious
behavior, and aggression that occur in some individuals. The use of *sign language*
is often helpful, especially for children who are non-verbal or who have very
limited verbal skills. Sign language is the process of using hand gestures to represent words. It can be used alone, or can be combined with verbalizations to
accompany the gestures, also commonly referred to as *signed speech, simultaneous*

communication, or *total communication*. Some children with autism learn more easily when using signed speech, while others have trouble associating auditory with visual symbols, and are best taught using sign alone. A subgroup of children with autism also have difficulty with learning to imitate motor patterns (called *dyspraxia*), and sign language may be too difficult for these children. Often, children who learn sign language are also provided with some sort of picture communications system so that they have a mechanism for communicating with people who do not know sign language. A trained speech-language therapist can provide insight as to the appropriateness of using sign language based on the individual learning profile of each child.

There are several different types of sign language. *American Sign Language* and *British Sign Language* are the languages typically used to teach children who are deaf. These languages use abbreviated syntax, such as saying "cup on table" to mean "the cup is on the table". Children with autism learn better when using a *signed English* method, where the signs represent exactly the same syntax as spoken language. This helps them to appreciate the normal conventions for grammar and syntax that are used during conversational speech. When sign language is used, it is helpful for all of the people who regularly work with the child to learn the signs, and to agree upon which aspects of communication to focus upon.

There is good research evidence to support the appropriateness of sign language for at least some children with autism, and to describe best practices in instruction when using this method. Sometimes, children will spontaneously develop verbal language once they have started to use signs, and the use of sign language can then be phased out to allow communication training using verbal strategies. Research also suggests that once children learn to communicate through signs, positive changes may also occur in eye contact, attention to others, and the ability to sit still during learning situations.

Training in sign language

The use of sign language to teach communication skills is typically provided by speech-language therapists who are regulated by their professional organizations, and who are best able to evaluate children to determine the appropriateness of using sign language as opposed to other types of intervention. Numerous opportunities exist for parents, teachers, and other therapists to learn sign language to provide follow-through of the instruction. This may occur through formal classes, workshops, or through reviewing books and videos.

Recommended resources for sign language

Literature

Bogdashina, O. (2004) *Communication Issues in Autism and Asperger Syndrome: Do we Speak the Same Language?* London: Jessica Kingsley Publishers.

Goldstein, H. (2002) 'Communication intervention for children with autism: A review of treatment efficacy.' *Journal of Autism and Developmental Disorders, 32,* 5, 373–396.

Mirenda, P. (2003) 'Toward a functional augmentative and alternate communication for students with autism: Manual signs, graphic symbols, and voice output communication aids.' *Language, Speech and Hearing Services in Schools, 34,* 203–216.

Seal, B.C. and Bonvillian, J.D. (1997) 'Sign language and motor functioning in students with autistic disorder.' *Journal of Autism and Developmental Disorders, 27,* 4, 437–466.

Schaeffer, B. (1980) 'Teaching signed speech to non-verbal children: Theory and method.' *Sign Language Studies, 26,* 29–63.

Vicker, B. (2001) 'Initial guidelines for developing a communication intervention plan for individuals with autism spectrum disorders and significant limitations in communication ability.' *The Reporter, 7,* 1, 18–25, 29.

Vicker, B. (2004) *Selected Bibliography: Communication Literature Related to Autism Spectrum Disorders.* Bloomington, IN: Indiana Resource Center for Autism.

Agencies, organizations, and websites

American Speech-Language Hearing Association (ASHA)

10801 Rockville Pike
Rockville, MD 20852, USA
Telephone: +1 (800) 638-8255
Website: www.asha.org
This is the professional, scientific and credentialing association for members and affiliates who are speech-language therapists, audiologists, and speech, language and hearing scientists in the United States.

National Institute on Deafness and Other Communication Disorders

National Institutes of Health
31 Center Drive, MSC 2320
Bethesda, MD 20892-2320, USA
Telephone: +1 (800) 241-1044
Website: www.nidcd.nih.gov

This organization maintains a directory of other organizations that can answer questions and provide printed or electronic information on autism and communication.

Royal College of Speech and Language Therapists
2 White Hart Yard
London SE1 1NX, UK
Telephone: +44 (0)207 378 1200
Website: www.rcslt.org
This organization represents speech and language therapists and support workers. It aims to promote excellence in practice, and to influence health, education, and social care policy.

SOCIAL STORIES™

The use of *Social Stories*™ is a concept developed by Carol Gray, who is a special education teacher specializing in working with children, adolescents, and adults with autism. Impairment with reciprocal social interaction is one of the diagnostic hallmarks of people with autism, because they fail to see and understand the perspective of another individual. Gray developed Social Stories™ as a way to help people with autism to better understand social situations and to appreciate the feelings and attitudes of others. Social Stories™ are developed according to the specific interests and problems of a particular child, for example learning to sit still in circle time, learning to stay calm during a fire drill, or learning to ask a friend to play a game. A story is then developed, written in the first person and present tense, and incorporating simple and clear descriptions of the social cues and appropriate behaviors that might occur in the particular situation. Because many children with autism are concrete, visual learners, the stories may be illustrated, recorded on videotape, or may use concrete objects as a prop. An adult then reads the story along with the child, asking questions or role-playing the situation to make sure the child understands the important elements of the social situation. The story is reviewed often, until the child demonstrates that he or she has mastered the skill and is generalizing the behaviors into daily life situations.

Gray recommends that stories be constructed using a specific pattern of sentences. It should start with several *descriptive sentences*, which describe what happens in a given situation. For example, in helping a child prepare to cope with a fire drill, the story might start with, "There is a loud bell at school that tells people when there is a real fire or when people need to practice getting out of the building in case of a fire. When the bell rings, everybody needs to line up. Then the teacher closes the door to the classroom, and helps all of the children to leave the school and line up outdoors. Her job is to make sure the children are safe. The bell is very loud and hurts my ears."

Next, the story offers some *perspective sentences*, which describe how different people might react to the situation. This helps the child to learn that others might react differently to the same situation. For example, "The loud bell frightens me, and makes me get nervous. Sometimes it makes me want to hide instead of leaving the school with the other children. Not everybody is afraid of the bell. The teacher gets frustrated if I don't do what I am supposed to do, because it is her job to make sure I am safe if there was ever a real fire."

Next, the story contains one or two *directive sentences* that teach the child a specific response to the situation. For example "I need to try hard to stay calm when the bell rings. It is OK to cover my ears, but I will try really hard to line up with the other children as soon as I hear the bell."

Finally, the story ends with *control sentences*. These are generated by the child, and describe strategies that will help the child to remember the important concepts in the story. For example, "When I hear the fire bell, I will think about the swings on the playground. I know that once I am outside and can see the swings, the noise won't bother me anymore."

The use of Social Stories™ has gained popularity, and there is growing evidence to support its effectiveness. It is a method that is easily incorporated into the therapy provided by teachers, psychologists, speech therapists, occupational therapists, and others who work with children with autism It is important for everyone who works with the child to know about each story as it is developed, so they can help to reinforce the concepts.

Training in Social Stories™

Continuing education workshops are available to psychologists, speech therapists, occupational therapists, parents, and others with an interest in learning to use Social Stories™. Many of the books about Social Stories™ also provide a very detailed description of the process so that the method can be self-taught at a relatively low cost.

Recommended resources for Social Stories™

Literature

Ali, S. and Frederickson, N. (2006) 'Investigating the evidence base of social stories.' *Educational Psychology in Practice, 22*, 4, 355–377.

Baker, J. (2003) *The Social Skills Picture Book: Teaching Play, Emotion, and Communication to Children with Autism.* Arlington, TX: Future Horizons, Inc.

Gray, C. (2000) *The New Social Story Book, Illustrated Edition.* Arlington, TX: Future Horizons, Inc.

Gray, C. and Leigh White, A. (eds.) (2001) *My Social Stories Book.* London: Jessica Kingsley Publishers.

Marr, D., Mika, H., Miraglia, J., Roerig, M. and Sinnott, R. (2007) 'The effects of sensory stories on targeted behaviors in preschool children with autism.' *Physical and Occupational Therapy in Pediatrics, 27*, 1, 63–79.

Scattione, D., Wilczynski, S.M. and Edwards, R.P. (2002) 'Decreasing disruptive behaviors of children using social stories.' *Journal of Autism and Developmental Disorders, 32*, 535–543.

Thieman, K.S. and Goldstein, H. (2001) 'Social stories, written text cues, and video feedback: Effects on social communication of children with autism.' *Journal of Applied Behavior Analysis, 34*, 425–446.

Agencies, organizations, and websites

The Gray Center for Social Learning and Understanding
4123 Embassy Drive, SE
Kentwood, MI 49546, USA
Telephone: +1 (616) 954-9747
Website: www.thegraycenter.org
This is Carol Gray's website. It offers information and guidelines about writing social stories, sample stories, and products for sale.

SON-RISE PROGRAM®

Son-Rise is a play-based treatment program that was developed during the late 1960s and the early 1970s by parents of a child with autism, Barry and Samahria Kaufman. The Kaufmans were unhappy with the medical advice they received for their child, and with the prognosis that autism is a serious and lifelong disorder. They chose to believe that children with autism engage in atypical behaviors, not because they have neurological differences affecting brain function, but because the behaviors serve some unknown purpose that is mean-ingful only to the child. In Son-Rise, parents and trained volunteers are taught to treat the child with a completely loving and accepting attitude, and to engage in whatever naturally occurring play that the child selects. They are taught to imitate the child in whatever behaviors are demonstrated, such as rocking, hand flapping, etc., and then to gradually introduce eye contact and communicative attempts during this play. The Kaufmans believe that the child with autism will sense the adult's attitude through voice tone and body language, and if the adult's attitude is one of accepting the child for who he or she is, the child will be encouraged to interact and communicate. The Kaufmans have written a number of books, and cite success with their son, Raun, who, according to them, became completely "normal", graduating from an Ivy League college and then working as an educational director for school-aged children.

There have been no formal research studies to prove the effectiveness of the Son-Rise Program®, although the Kaufmans have collected parent satisfaction data that suggests improvements in language acquisition, eye contact, and attention span. Critics question whether the program offers false hope to parents, and express concern about the cost and intensive nature of the program.

Training in the Son-Rise Program™

The Autism Center of America™ offers several non-certification and certification training programs for parents and others with an interest in learning about the Son-Rise Program®. The Son-Rise Program® Child Facilitator program teaches students to work directly with children and adults with autism, and takes 18 months to complete. The Son-Rise Program® Instructor Certification focuses on the leadership and communication skills needed to work with parents and volunteers, and takes an additional 24 months for completion. Instructors who have completed this level of certification may be employed by the Autism Treatment Center of America™ or may develop a private practice.

Recommended resources for the Son-Rise Program™

Literature

Kaufman, B.N and Kaufman, R. (1995) *Son-Rise: The Miracle Continues*. Tiburon, CA: H.J. Kramer, Inc.

Kaufman, B.N. (1994) *Happiness is a Choice*. New York: Ballantine Books.

Williams, K.R. (2006) 'The Son-Rise Program® intervention for autism: Prerequisites for evaluation.' *Autism, 10*, 1, 86–102.

Williams, K.R. and Wishart, J.G. (2003) 'The Son-Rise Program® intervention for autism: An investigation into family experiences.' *Journal of Intellectual Disability Research, 47*, pt 4–5, 291–299.

Agencies, organizations, and websites
Autism Treatment Center of America™
The Son-Rise Program® at the Options Institute
2080 S. Undermountain Road
Sheffield, MA 01257, USA

Telephone: +1 (413) 229-2100

Website: www.autismtreatmentcenter.org

This is the worldwide teaching center for the Son-Rise Program®, offering information, products, and training programs and packages.

TEACCH

TEACCH (Treatment and Education of Autistic and Related Communication Handicapped Children) is part of the Department of Psychiatry, School of Medicine, at the University of North Carolina at Chapel Hill. Developed in the early 1970s by psychologist Eric Schopler, it is a comprehensive statewide program of education and advocacy that aims to help people with autism of all ages to live and work more effectively at home, in school, and in the community. Central to the philosophy of TEACCH is a respect for the unique culture of "being autistic". Rather than attempting to make people with autism conform to some predetermined concept of "normality", people with autism are guided to develop their own unique potential. Several key concepts are important to the TEACCH model. First, it uses a highly structured educational environment that includes organizing the physical environment for predictability, making clear expectations, and providing explicit, visually designed schedules. Regularly scheduled *Psychoeducational Profiles (PEP)* are conducted to make sure that the program is individually tailored to changing needs. Parents are regarded as "co-therapists" and are considered an important part of the team effort. Behavioral strategies emphasize meaningful functional rewards instead of tokens or food rewards. Finally, the program places a strong emphasis on identifying the individual's unique skills and interests, and building on these instead of focusing only on remediating areas of deficit. TEACCH is a very broad-based program that is believed to work because of its deep understanding and respect for the culture of autism. It does not have specific methodologies or protocols that can be taught, per se, to others. People who are taught through TEACCH continuing education programs are considered to be generalists who understand the whole person, as opposed to professionals with a narrow interest in one aspect of function, such as speech or behavior. TEACCH, as it was developed, is not available as a comprehensive program outside of the state of North Carolina in the United States. However, training is available to teach some of the philosophy and methods to professionals in other countries.

Training in TEACCH

The Division of TEACCH at the University of North Carolina at Chapel Hill offers a number of continuing education opportunities to learn more about this particular philosophy. There is no formal mechanism for certification or registration as a practitioner of this approach.

Recommended resources for TEACCH
Literature

Mesibov, G.B., Shea, V. and Schopler, E. (2005) *The TEACCH Approach to Autism Spectrum Disorders.* New York: Springer Publishers.

Mesibov, G.B. and Howley, M. (2005) *Accessing the Curriculum for Pupils with Autism Spectrum Disorder.* London: David Fulton Publishers.

Panerai, S., Ferrante, L. and Zingale, M. (2002) 'Benefits of the Treatment and Education of Autistic and Communication Handicapped Children (TEACCH) programme as compared with a non-specific approach.' *Journal of Intellectual Disability Research, 46,* 4, 318–327.

Panerai, S., Ferrante, L. and Caputo, V. (1997) 'The TEACCH strategy in mentally retarded children with autism: A multidimensional assessment. Pilot study. Treatment and Education of Autistic and Communication Handicapped Children.' *Journal of Autism and Developmental Disorders, 27,* 3, 345–347.

Agencies, organizations, and websites
Division TEACCH
Department of Psychiatry, School of Medicine
University of North Carolina at Chapel Hill
Chapel Hill, NC 27599-7180, USA
Telephone: +1 (919) 966-2174
Website: www.teacch.com
This is the official website of the TEACCH program which offers service, research, and training for persons with autism and their families.

The National Autistic Society
393 City Road
London EC1V 1NG, UK
Telephone: +44 (0)207 833 2299
Website: www.nas.org.uk
Further information about TEACCH in the UK can be found at this website.

TRANSCENDENTAL MEDITATION

Meditation refers to a variety of techniques that have been promoted for centuries, largely by Buddhist monks, as way to induce a relaxed state for the purpose of developing inner peace and harmony. *Transcendental meditation* is one form of meditation that was first popularized about 50 years ago by Maharishi Mahesh

Yogi, and is often practiced in conjunction with Ayurvedic methods of health care. It has attracted recent interest as a possible method for helping children with ADHD, Asperger's syndrome, or mood disorders to improve in the areas of impulsiveness, hyperactivity, and inattention. Proponents of transcendental meditation describe it as a simple, natural technique that involves posing in a relaxing position, focusing on specialized breathing techniques, and repeating a chant, also called a *mantra*, to induce relaxation and inner awareness. Adults usually sit still with their eyes closed for 20 minutes and repeat a familiar mantra such as *"om"*, but for children, the techniques are different. Although some children may be able to sit still, many need to do their mediation while walking to school or playing quietly. The use of visualization and more child-friendly mantras helps young children to stay focused and relaxed. Children also meditate for shorter periods of time than adults. Some schools promote daily meditation for all students, including those without disabilities, as a method for promoting relaxation and decreasing stress. Limited scientific research has been conducted to determine the effectiveness of meditation as a specific intervention for children with disabilities.

Training in transcendental meditation

Meditation is a tool that is used by many teachers, therapists, psychologists, and others, and its practice is not regulated in either the United States or the United Kingdom. There are numerous continuing education opportunities for learning mediation techniques, and advanced training is available through universities that include meditation training as part of a more comprehensive program in holistic health education. Meditation techniques can also be self-taught, and there are many books and videos that can serve as a guide.

Recommended resources for transcendental meditation

Literature

Canter, P.H. and Ernst, E. (2003) 'The cumulative effects of Transcendental Meditation on cognitive function: A systematic review of randomized controlled trials.' *Wiener Klinische Wochenschrift, 115*, 21–22, 758–766.

Desmond, L. (2004) *Baby Buddhas: A Guide for Teaching Meditation to Children.* Riverside, NJ: Andrews McMeel Publishing.

Fontina, D. (2002) *Teaching Meditation to Children: A Practical Guide to the Use and Benefits of Meditation.* Wellingborough, UK: Thorsons Publishing Group.

Rozman, D. (2002) *Meditating with Children – The Art of Concentration and Centering: A Workbook on New Educational Methods Using Meditation.* Buckingham, VA: Integral Yoga Publications.

Agencies, organizations, and websites

Maharishi School of the Age of Enlightenment
Cobbs Brow Lane, Lathom
Ormskirk L40 6JJ, UK
Telephone: +44 (0)1695 729912
Website: www.maharishischool.com
This is an independent school that incorporates transcendental meditation and creative intelligence into its curriculum.

Maharishi University of Management
Fairfield, IA 52557, USA
Telephone: +1 (641) 472-7000
Website: www.mum.edu
This university offers undergraduate and graduate degrees in the arts, sciences, business, and humanities with a focus on transcendental meditation.

Transcendental Meditation Organization
Telephone: +1 (888) 532 7686 (USA)
            +44 (0)8705 14373 (UK)
Website: www.tm.org (USA)
            www.transcendental-meditation.org.uk (UK)
These websites provide general information pertaining to transcendental meditation, and offer links to programs that offer training in the techniques endorsed by Maharishi Mahesh Yogi.

Transcendental Meditation
24 Linhope Street
London NW1 6HT, UK
Telephone: +44 (0)207 402 3787
Website: www.tm-london.org.uk
This is a local organization providing information and resources about transcendental meditation.

VIDEO MODELING

Video modeling is a specialized teaching method that can produce rapid learning of a variety of skills in children, especially those with autism spectrum disorders. It involves presenting the child with a videotaped sample of how to behave in certain selected social situations. Video modelling may be used to teach children how to play, how to perform self-care activities, how to communicate in social situations, or how to behave appropriately under challenging circumstances.

The method involves choosing a specific behavior that the child needs to learn, such as how to initiate and hold a conversation with peers. A videotape is produced using "actors" who model the situation (for example, holding a conversation) using scripted actions and verbalizations. The child then watches the videotape, and practices using the scripted actions and verbalizations until he or she can carry them out in a real life situation. In some cases, especially with children who are higher functioning, the child actually participates in developing the script according to some personal aspiration, and then becomes the actor in his or her own videotape. Because many children with autism are attracted to visual stimuli such as those involved in watching a videotape, they tend to be more motivated to attend to these lessons. Research has shown that children with autism are more likely to learn from video modeling than from live modeling, where a live person acts out the behavior. Video modeling is commonly used as part of a treatment regimen that incorporates principles of *applied behavior analysis*. As such, various prompting and reinforcement strategies are often used to ensure that the child learns and generalizes the skills that are being taught through watching the videotape.

Training in video modeling

Video modeling techniques may be learned through a variety of ways. It is often included in the professional curriculum of psychologists and other professionals who learn applied behavior analysis methods as part of their curriculum. Numerous workshops, continuing education seminars, on-line courses, and books also provide opportunities for professionals from a range of disciplines to learn the techniques.

Recommended resources for video modeling

Literature

Bellini, S. and Akullian, J. (2007) 'A meta-analysis of video modeling and video self-modeling interventions for children and adolescents with autism spectrum disorders.' *Exceptional Children, 73*, 3, 264–288.

Charlop-Christy, M.H., Le, L. and Freeman, K.A. (2000) 'A comparison of video modeling with in vivo modeling for teaching children with autism.' *Journal of Autism and Developmental Disorders, 30*, 6, 537–552.

Charlop, M.H. and Milstein, J.P. (1989) 'Teaching autistic children conversational speech using video modeling.' *Journal of Applied Behavior Analysis, 22*, 3, 275–285.

Corbett, B.A. and Abdullah, M. (2005) 'Video modeling: Why does it work for children with autism?' *Journal of Early Intensive Behavioral Intervention, 2,* 2–8.

Hitchcock, C.H., Dowrick, P.W. and Prater, M.A. (2006) 'Video self-modeling in school-based settings: A review.' *Remedial and Special Education, 24,* 1, 36–46.

Neuman, L. (2004) *Video Modeling: A Visual Teaching Method for Children with Autism.* Brandon, FL: Willerik Publishing.

Nikopoulos, C.K. and Keenan, M. (2007) 'Using video modeling to teach complex social sequences to children with autism.' *Journal of Autism and Developmental Disorders, 37,* 4, 678–693.

Nikopoulos, C.K. and Keenan, M. (2004) 'Effects of video modeling on social initiations by children with autism.' *Journal of Applied Behavior Analysis, 37,* 1, 93–96.

Nikopoulos, C.K. and Keenan, M. (2006) *Video Modelling and Behaviour Analysis: A Guide for Teaching Social Skills to Children with Autism.* London: Jessica Kingsley Publishers.

Agencies, organizations, and websites

Association for Behavior Analysis International

1219 South Park Street
Kalamazoo, MI 49001, USA
Telephone: +1 (269) 492-9310
Website: www.abainternational.org
This is the primary professional organization for members interested in the philosophy, science, application, and teaching of behavior analysis. It provides information about research and educational resources, opportunities for training, and publications pertaining to applied behavior analysis.

Interactive Collaborative Autism Network

Website: www.autismnetwork.org
This website offers a good introduction and "hands-on" guide to the use of video modeling in children with autism and other developmental disabilities. It also offers a series of on-line instructional modules about autism spectrum disorders and various intervention methods.

Chapter 5

BIOLOGICALLY-BASED INTERVENTIONS

BACH FLOWER REMEDIES

Bach flower remedies are a type of homeopathic intervention developed in the 1930s by British physician Edward Bach to help to manage behaviors associated with stress and anxiety. They are sometimes used to help children with agitation or anxiety related to autism or ADHD. Through a largely intuitive process of self-discovery, Bach identified 38 flower essences that he believed could affect specific moods. The essences are derived by steeping flowers in water that is exposed to sunlight, or by boiling the flowers, to create a *mother tincture*. This tincture is then diluted before its use. To use the essences, the tincture is further diluted with water, along with brandy, alcohol, or vinegar added as a preservative, and is then taken orally, or occasionally as a salve to rub into the skin. The amount of the essence used is extremely small, so that there is no recognizable flavor or taste of the original flower. Essences may be taken alone, or in combinations that are created to address specific emotional or behavioral concerns. For example, the most commonly marketed essence is called *Rescue Remedy,* which is a combination of five remedies designed to treat stress, anxiety, and panic attacks. Because there has been little scientific inquiry as to the effectiveness of these remedies, their use is not generally supported by the mainstream medical community, although they remain popular among consumers as a natural alternative to traditional therapies.

Training in Bach flower remedies

The Dr Edward Bach Foundation, sponsored through the Bach Centre in England, sponsors three levels of training for practitioners interested in using the essences. Other organizations sponsor continuing education programs and develop essences in the tradition of Bach. The use of flower essences is not formally regulated in either the United States or the United Kingdom, although producers of the essences must meet governmental standards of production, ensuring safety and approved labeling. Many consumers of flower essences are self-taught, and purchase the remedies through health food stores and suppliers.

Recommended resources for Bach flower remedies

Literature

Bach, E. (1998) *The Bach Flower Remedies*. New York: McGraw Hill.

Ernst, E. (2002) 'Flower remedies: A systematic review of the clinical evidence.' *Wiener Klinische Wochenschrift, 114*, 23–24, 963–966.

Monovoisin, R. (2005) 'Bach flower remedies: A critic of the pseudoscientific, pseudomedicinal concepts and philosophical postures inducted by Dr. Bach theory.' *Annales Pharmaceutiques Francaises, 63*, 6, 416–428.

Pintiv, S., Hochman, M., Livine, A., Heyman, E. and Lahat, E. (2005) 'Bach flower remedies used for attention deficit hyperactivity disorder in children: A prospective double blind controlled study.' *European Journal of Paediatric Neurology, 9*, 6, 395–398.

Agencies, organizations, and websites

Dr Edward Bach Centre
Mount Vernon, Bakers Lane
Brightwell-cum-Sotwell, Oxon OX10 0PZ, UK
Telephone: +44 (0)1491 834678
Website: www.bachcentre.com
This website offers information, training, and references about flower remedies, as well as an extensive international listing of registered practitioners.

Flower Essences Society
PO Box 459
Nevada City, CA 95959, USA
Telephone:+1 (800) 736-9222 (toll-free from within US and Canada)
          +1 (530) 265-9163
Website: www.flowersociety.org
This is an international membership organization of health practitioners, researchers, and others interested in flower essence therapy. It conducts training and certification programs, as well as offering a referral network.

The British Association of Flower Essence Producers
PO Box 100
Exminster, Exeter, Devon EX6 8YT, UK
Telephone: +44 (0)1392 832005
Website: www.bafep.com

This is the trade organization for producers of Bach flower remedies and other types of essences. It sets and maintains standards of production, labeling, and advertising in accordance with the guidelines of various UK governmental agencies.

CHELATION THERAPY

Chelation therapy is a chemical method for removing heavy metal toxins from the bloodstream through intravenous injections, or occasionally through the use of orally administered or *transdermally* (through the skin) administered substances. The most commonly used chelating agent is an organic chemical called *ethylene diamine tetra-acedic (EDTA)*, which is a man-made amino acid that attracts such metals as mercury, lead, aluminum, and cadmium. Chelation therapy is the treatment of choice for known poisonings with metals such as lead. More recently, it has gained attention as a possible treatment for children with autism, ADHD, and language learning disorders. Some researchers believe that children with autism show evidence of poisoning from heavy metals, especially mercury, that are continuously present in our environment. In particular, there has been concern that some children have developed symptoms of autism after having received vaccinations during early childhood that have contained the mercury-based preservative, *thimerosal*, which is present in some vaccines. Although blood and hair sample studies have failed to show that children with autism have clinical evidence of mercury toxicity, proponents of this theory believe that for individuals with detoxification abnormalities, the mercury binds to enzymes and proteins in the liver, kidney, brain, and other organs so that little remains in the hair or bloodstream, producing false-negative test results.

Chelation therapy for neurodevelopmental disorders has been heavily criticized by the mainstream medical community, as extensive studies have revealed no evidence of a link between mercury exposure and autism, and because it is considered a potentially unsafe intervention. In some cases, the treatment can lead to serious, or even potentially fatal, liver or kidney failure. In addition, because the chelating agents are not specific to mercury, they also remove other essential mineral nutrients, such as calcium, zinc, and iron, which must then be carefully replaced to maintain health. The intravenous procedure typically requires multiple treatments, each lasting for several hours, and is not usually covered by health insurance. Advocates present anecdotal claims that chelation therapy effectively reduces many symptoms of childhood autism, especially among younger children who experienced a history of normal development followed by regression of development leading to autism. As thimerosal has been removed from most childhood vaccines in both the United States and the

United Kingdom, some proponents are looking to see if the incidence of autism declines.

Training in chelation therapy

Chelation therapy is a medical procedure that must be carried out by a trained physician, since serious adverse effects can occur. Several deaths have been reported among children undergoing intravenous chelation, so this is a treatment that must be considered only with extreme caution.

Recommended resources for chelation therapy

Literature

Andrews, N., Miller, E., Grant, A., Stowe, J., Osborne, V. and Taylor, B. (2004) 'Thimerosal exposure in infants and developmental disorders: A retrospective cohort study in the United Kingdom does not support a causal association.' *Pediatrics, 114*, 3, 584–591.

Doja, A. and Roberts, W. (2006) 'Immunizations and autism: A review of the literature.' *Canadian Journal of Neurological Sciences, 33*, 4, 341–346.

Green, J. (2006) 'Overview: Detoxification through chelation therapy.' *Autism Research Review International: 20*, 1, 3.

Honda, H., Shimizu, Y. and Rutter, M. (2005) 'No effect of MMR withdrawal on the incidence of autism: A total population study.' *Journal of Child Psychology and Psychiatry, 46*, 572–579.

Hviid, A., Stellfield, M., Wohlfahrt, J. and Melbye, M. (2003) 'Association between thimerosal-containing vaccine and autism.' *Journal of the American Medical Association, 290*, 13, 1763–1766.

Immunization Safety Review Committee (2004) *Immunization Safety Review: Vaccines and Autism.* Washington, DC: Institute of Medicine.

Nelson, K.B. and Bauman, M.L. (2003) 'Thimerosal and autism?' *Pediatrics, 111*, 674–679.

Ng, D.K., Chan, C.H., Soo, M.T. and Lee, R.S. (2007) 'Low-level chronic mercury exposure in children and adolescents: Meta-analysis.' *Pediatrics International: Official Journal of the Japan Pediatrics Society, 49*, 1, 80–87.

Parker, S.K., Schwartz, B., Todd, J. and Pickering, L.K. (2004) 'Thimerosal-containing vaccines and autistic spectrum disorder: A critical review of published original data.' *Pediatrics, 114*, 3, 793–804.

Agencies, organizations, and websites

Centers for Disease Control and Prevention

1600 Clifton Road

Atlanta, GA 30333, USA

Telephone: +1 (800) 311-3435

Website: www.cdc.gov

This official agency of the United States government offers recommendations about childhood immunizations, including information about current research into the possible link between vaccines and autism.

Generation Rescue

Website: www.generationrescue.org

This is a parent-funded and parent-led organization that promotes the dissemination of information about mercury poisoning in children with autism.

National Library for Health

Website: www.library.nhs.uk

This is a service of the National Health Service in the United Kingdom, and offers free full-text versions of many helpful articles relating to the relationship between autism and vaccines.

National Vaccine Information Center

204 Mill Street, Suite B1

Vienna, VA 22180, USA

Telephone: +1 (703) 938-0342

Website: www.909shot.com

This is a national, non-profit educational organization advocating the institution of vaccine safety and informed consent protections for vaccination programs in the United States.

CRANIAL ELECTROTHERAPY STIMULATION (CES)

Cranial electrotherapy stimulation (CES) is the use of low intensity microcurrent (under one milliampere) to stimulate various parts of the brain in an effort to achieve neurochemical changes as an alternative to drug therapy. It is widely used as a treatment for insomnia, depression, and anxiety, but has also been proposed as an alternative intervention for children with autism and ADHD. Cranial electrotherapy stimulation is also known by several other terms, including *transcranial electrotherapy, microcurrent electrical therapy, electromedical treatment,* and *electrosleep.* This treatment is non-invasive, and involves placing electrodes on or near the ear while a hand-held device produces the electrical current that travels to the brain. Various protocols exist, but typically the stimulation is provided daily for a period of two to three weeks, and is then provided on a less frequent basis. Children are able to read, watch television, or listen to music during the therapy. Effects are generally immediate, but are also cumulative, so it is important to maintain the recommended protocol to achieve the full benefits of the therapy.

The theory behind CES is that the microcurrent travels to the brainstem and activates nerve cells that produce the neurotransmitters *serotonin* and *acetylcholine*. These chemicals are linked to relaxation and to the inhibition of arousal and agitation. Their release is believed to help the brain to create an *alpha wave rhythm*, which promotes mental focus and relaxation.

Patients often describe the sensation of CES to be pleasant, and to help them to immediately feel relaxed and more mentally alert. They often report a tingling or pulsing sensation in the earlobe which is not painful. Side effects are few, and may include mild headaches, lightheadedness, or skin irritation from the electrodes. Rarely, more serious side effects have been reported, including sleep disturbances, excessive excitement, or an increase in anxiety.

In the United States, the Federal Food and Drug Administration (FDA) approves cranial electrotherapy stimulation for the treatment of insomnia, depression, and anxiety, but not for other medical conditions including pain management, chemical dependency, autism or ADHD. Because physicians are not typically trained in its use, and continuing education opportunities are limited, this treatment is often recommended by psychologists or alternative health providers who may not have a full understanding of the medical and neuropsychological implications of these conditions. Critics express concern that CES treatment focuses on alleviating a set of symptoms, rather than treating the underlying condition.

Training in cranial electrotherapy stimulation

This intervention is not typically included in the professional curriculum for physicians. Most practitioners receive post-graduate training through continuing education seminars that are offered by the manufacturers of the devices used in the treatment.

Recommended resources for cranial electrotherapy stimulation

Literature

Kirsch, D.L. and Giordano, J. (2006) 'Cranial electrotherapy.' *Natural Medicine*, *23*, 118–120.

Klawansky, S., Yeung, A., Berkey, C., Shah, N., Phan, H. and Chalmers, T.C. (1995) 'Meta-analysis of randomized controlled trial of cranial electrostimulation: Efficacy in treating selected psychological and physiological conditions.' *Journal of Nervous and Mental Diseases*, 7, 478–484.

Overcash, S. (2005) 'The effect of ROSHI protocol and cranial electrotherapy stimulation on a 9-year-old anxious, dyslexic male with attention deficit disorder: A case study.' *Journal of Neurotherapy*, 9, 2, 63–77.

Smith, R.B. (2002) 'Microcurrent therapies: Emerging theories of physiological information processing.' *Neurorehabilitation*, 17, 1, 3–7.

Southworth, S. (1999) 'A study of the effects of cranial electrical stimulation on attention and concentration.' *Integrative Physiological and Behavioral Science: The Official Journal of the Pavlovian Society*, 34, 1, 43–53.

Agencies, organizations, and websites
Electromedical Products International, Inc.
2201 Garret Morris Parkway
Mineral Wells, TX 76067-9034, USA
Telephone: +1 (940) 328-0788
Website: www.alpha-stim.com
This is the company that produces the Alpha-Stim® cranial electrotherapy stimulation technology, which is one of the most commonly used devices worldwide. In addition to offering product sales and information, it provides general information and references relating to CES.

DAN! PROTOCOL

DAN stands for *Defeat Autism Now*, which is a project of the Autism Research Institute (ARI), founded by psychologist and child advocate Bernard Rimland and his associates in the late 1960s. Dr Rimland had a son with autism, and was frustrated by the lack of medical interventions available for the condition. As a result, he and his associates began investigating various theories about the cause(s) of autism as well as the potential of various biomedical interventions. Proponents of this approach believe that there are several causes of autism that are not well accepted by the mainstream medical community. These may include a genetic predisposition to certain conditions, mercury poisoning, viral infections secondary to certain infant immunizations, food allergies, a compromised immune system, excessive yeast in the digestive tract, reactions to antibiotics, or a lack of (or poor absorption of) certain key nutrients. Their ongoing research eventually led to the development of the DAN! Protocol. This usually involves extensive testing, usually including allergy tests and laboratory analysis of hair and nail clippings to determine mercury levels. Following this analysis, a DAN doctor will develop a personalized biomedical treatment plan which often involves a number of non-conventional medical treatments, often including nutritional supplements, chelation therapy, gluten-free or dairy-free diets, and treatment of yeast infections with probiotics. These interventions are usually combined with other more traditional treatments, including applied behavior analysis and special education intervention. Critics of the DAN! Protocol cite concern about the poor reliability of certain types of testing, and caution parents that some of the interventions have the potential to cause serious side effects.

Training in the DAN! Protocol

A one-day training seminar is offered by the Autism Research Institute (ARI) to credentialed medical doctors who are interested in learning about the DAN! Protocol. For doctors who are interested in becoming registered with the ARI as a doctor who follows the DAN! methods, the ARI requires them to attend a seminar at least once every two years to stay current with the latest research and methods. The ARI does not, however, investigate the qualifications of doctors who attend their seminars, so consumers are cautioned to investigate the credentials and expertise of any practitioner who claims to be knowledgeable about the DAN! Protocol.

Recommended resources for the DAN! Protocol

Literature

Baker, S.M. (2003) *Detoxification and Healing: The Key to Optimal Health*. Los Angeles, CA: Keats Publishing Company.

Levy, S.E. and Hyman, S.L. (2003) 'Use of complementary and alternative treatments for children with autism spectrum disorders is increasing.' *Pediatric Annals*, *32*, 10, 685–691.

McCandless, J. (2007) *Children with Starving Brains: A Medical Treatment Guide for Autism Spectrum Disorders, 3rd edn*. Putney, VT: Bramble Books.

Pangborn, J. and Baker, S.M. (2005) *Autism: Effective Biomedical Treatments (Have We Done Everything We Can for This Child? Individuality in an Epidemic), 2nd edn*. San Diego, CA: Autism Research Institute.

Agencies, organizations, and websites

Autism Research Institute (ARI)

4182 Adams Avenue
San Diego, CA 92116, USA
Fax: +1 (619) 563-6840

Website: www.autism.com
This is the homepage for the ARI. It offers information about biomedical
treatments for autism, links to upcoming seminars, and an international registry
of doctors trained in the DAN! Protocol.

DIETARY SUPPLEMENTS

Dietary supplements include vitamins, minerals, fatty acids, or amino acids that are
believed to be missing or insufficiently consumed in a person's diet. They may
also include herbal remedies that are thought to prevent or treat certain diseases
or conditions. There are numerous supplements that have gained popularity as
potential treatments for children with autism, ADHD, or other learning disabilities. Some of the more common ones are summarized in this section. All of
these interventions are considered experimental at this time, and should not be
considered without appropriate advice from a qualified physician.

Secretin is a natural protein hormone that is found in the liver, pancreas, intes-
tines, and brain. It may be administered either through intravenous injection or
through the skin (*transdermal*) in an effort to stimulate the pancreas to release
enzymes that might help to break down certain proteins. There is limited
research to show effectiveness, but anecdotal reports suggest that some children
will show improvement in gastrointestinal symptoms, with resulting improvements in cognitive and behavioral function. Alternatively, some people advocate
the use of supplemental digestive enzymes that may help to break down
proteins in the intestinal tract.

Multivitamin and mineral supplements are often used in an effort to improve the
immune system. Various supplements may be recommended, especially vitamin
B15 (also called *dimethylglycine (DMG), or pantothenic acid)* which is a naturally-
occurring amino acid, or vitamin B6 (*pyroxidine*) combined with magnesium.
These are believed to be beneficial in improving attention, learning and eye
contact. There is also evidence that vitamin B6 combined with magnesium may
help to reduce seizure activity, to decrease self-stimulation, and to improve
speech. Other popular supplements include vitamins A, B3, C, and folic acid;
and the minerals calcium, iron, and zinc.

Abnormal levels of *essential fatty acids* have also been implicated in the behavioral and learning problems seen in children with autism, ADHD, and dyslexia.
These fatty acids play an important role in the body's metabolism, nervous
system function, and ability to fight inflammation. They are also important in
certain aspects of visual functioning and in regulating stress. Essential fatty
acids are the healthy polyunsaturated fats that help to improve cardiovascular
health when they are used to replace saturated fats. There are two groups of fatty

acids. *Omega-6 fatty* acids are found in certain grains, meat, milk, eggs and corn oil. *Omega-3 fatty acids* are found primarily in oily fish, such as tuna, sardines, salmon, and mackerel, but are also found in walnuts and canola oil. These substances cannot be produced by the body, so it is critical that the diet contains enough of these substances to maintain a healthy balance. Supplementation may take the form of eating foods rich in essential fatty acids, or taking pills or fish oils by mouth.

Melatonin is a hormone that is secreted by the pineal gland in the brain. It responds to the natural changes in light that occur during the day, and helps people sleep by stabilizing their biological rhythms. It is also believed to help alleviate certain types of anxiety and depression. Melatonin levels are naturally higher at night, and begin to diminish as daylight increases. Studies have shown that some people with autism have deficient levels of melatonin. Melatonin supplementation may be used for short-term help with alertness and sleeplessness in children with autism and related disorders, but long-term use may alter biologic rhythms in a negative way.

L-carnosine is a synthetic version of a natural antioxidant protein that is normally found in the tissues of the heart, muscles, and brain. It affects the frontal part of the brain which controls emotion, seizure activity, cognition, speech, and abstract reasoning, and acts to reduce the production of abnormal proteins. L-carnosine has been well established as an anti-aging nutrient and is used in the treatment of such diseases as cancer, cataracts, and Alzheimer's disease. Some studies suggest that it shows potential for improving the language and behavior of children with autism, especially when taken in combination with other antioxidants such as zinc and vitamin E.

Probiotics are supplements that are used to help restore healthy levels of digestive bacteria that may have been disrupted through the use of antibiotic therapy. Most people are familiar with the gastric discomfort that is often correlated with taking antibiotics. Some researchers believe that some children with autism have depressed immune systems, leading to frequent ear infections and other problems requiring the use of antibiotics. These children seem to be unusually susceptible to yeast infections, which may interfere with the ability of the intestine to break down certain proteins. Because yeasts thrive on sugar, many parents attempt to control yeast infections by limiting the intake of dietary sugars and foods containing yeasts. Others supplement the diet with digestive enzymes, foods that fight yeasts such as yogurt, grape-seed oil or garlic, or helpful bacteria such as *lactobacillus acidophilus* or *bifidobacterium bifidum*. Occasionally, doctors may recommend the use of antifungal medications such as *Nystatin* or *Diflucan*.

Herbal supplements are widely used throughout the world for their potential therapeutic or medicinal benefits. Some, such as *kava kava* and *valerian* are believed to help to reduce stress and anxiety. *Gingko biloba* is commonly used to promote the flow of blood to the brain, and may help with some aspects of memory and learning. Some, including *aloe vera gel, chamomile, licorice,* and *sasparilla* may help to reduce stomach irritation and calm the nerves. Several herbs are believed to have antiseptic or antibiotic properties. Some of the more familiar of these include *echinacea purpurea, bitter melon,* and *goldenseal.*

Risperidone is an atypical antipsychotic drug that is commonly used in the treatment of serious psychiatric conditions. It is considered effective, usually in small doses, to reduce irritability, aggressiveness, and self-injurious behavior in children with autism spectrum disorders. There are a number of potentially serious side effects, so the use of this medication requires close medical supervision. Also, approximately one-third of children experience significant weight gain, which may limit its usefulness for long-term therapy.

Training in dietary supplements

Most dietary supplements are readily available to consumers who wish to try these products, although their cost may be prohibitive. They may be commonly found in supermarkets, pharmacies and health food stores, and are also available online through a variety of sources. They should be used with caution as significant side effects are possible, especially when taken in combination with certain foods, medications, or other supplements. In addition, consumers should be aware that dietary supplements are not regulated in the same way as medications. That means that dietary supplements can be sold even if there is no documented research to support the potential benefits. In the United States, the Food and Drug Administration (FDA) regulates dietary supplements as foods, and does not regulate their safety or efficacy in the same way as medications. The FDA can only intervene if a supplement proves to have harmful effects. In Europe, the Food Supplements Directive of 2002 requires supplements to be safe both in quality and quantity if they are to be sold without a prescription. Parents are strongly encouraged to discuss all options with their pediatrician before introducing any new dietary supplement.

Recommended resources for dietary supplements

Literature

Adams, J.B. and Holloway, C. (2004) 'Pilot study of a moderate dose
    multivitamin/mineral supplement for children with autism spectrum
    disorder.' *Journal of Alternative and Complementary Medicine, 10,* 6, 1033–1039.

Barrett, B., Kiefer, D. and Rabago, D. (1999) 'Assessing the risks and benefits of herbal medicine: An overview of scientific evidence.' *Alternative Therapies in Health and Medicine, 5*, 4, 40–49.

Chez, M.G., Buchanan, C.P., Aimonovitch, M.C., *et al.* (2002) 'Double-blind, placebo-controlled study of l-carnosine supplementation in children with autism spectrum disorders.' *Journal of Child Neurology, 17*, 11, 833–837.

Esch, B.E. and Carr, J.E. (2004) 'Secretin as a treatment for autism: A review of the evidence.' *Journal of Autism and Developmental Disorders, 34*, 5, 543–556.

Kidd, P.M. (2002) 'Autism, an extreme challenge to integrative medicine. Part 1: The knowledge base.' *Alternative Medicine Review, 7*, 4, 292–316.

Kidd, P.M. (2002) 'Autism, an extreme challenge to integrative medicine. Part 2: Medical management.' *Alternative Medicine Review, 7*, 6, 472–499.

Konofal, E., Lecendreux, M., Arnulf, I. and Mouren, M.C. (2004) 'Iron deficiency in children with attention deficit hyperactivity disorder.' *Archives of Pediatric and Adolescent Medicine, 158*, 1113–1115.

Levy, S.E. and Hyman, S.L. (2005) 'Novel treatments for autism spectrum disorders.' *Mental Retardation and Developmental Disabilities Research Review, 11*, 2 , 131–142.

Marohn, S. (2002) *The Natural Medicine Guide to Autism.* Charlottesville, VA: Hampton Roads Publishing Co.

McCandless, J. (2005) *Children with Starving Brains: A Medical Treatment Guide for Autism Spectrum Disorders, 2nd edn.* Putney, VT: Bramble Books.

Nye, C. and Brice, A. (2005) 'Combined vitamin B6-magnesium treatment in autism spectrum disorder.' *Cochrane Database Systematic Reviews, Oct. 19, 4,* CD003497.

Physician's Desk Reference (PDR) (2006) *PDR for Nonprescription Drugs, Dietary Supplements and Herbs: The Definitive Guide to OTC Medication, 27th edn.* Montvale, NJ: Thomson Healthcare.

Research Units on Pediatric Psychopharmacology Autism Network (2005) 'Risperidone treatment of autistic disorder: Longer-term benefits and blinded discontinuation after 6 months.' *American Journal of Psychiatry, 162*, 7, 1361–1369.

Richardson, A.J. and Montgomery, P. (2005) 'The Oxford-Durham study: A randomized controlled trial of dietary supplementation with fatty acids in children with developmental coordination disorder.' *Pediatrics, 115,* 5, 1360–1366.

Troost, P.W., Lahuis, B.E., Steenhuis, M.P., *et al.* (2005) 'Long-term effects of risperidone in children with autism spectrum disorders: A placebo discontinuation study.' *Journal of the American Academy of Child and Adolescent Psychiatry, 44*, 11, 1137–1144.

Williams, K.W., Wray, J.J. and Wheeler, D.M. (2005) 'Intravenous secretin for autism spectrum disorder.' *Cochrane Database Systematic Reviews, July 20, 3,* CD003495.

Agencies, organizations, and websites

Autism Research Unit (ARU)
School of Health, Natural & Social Sciences
City Campus, University of Sunderland
Sunderland SR1 3SD, UK
Telephone: +44 (0)191 567 0420
Website: http://www.osiris.sunderland.ac.uk/autism
This website offers information about various biomedical interventions for the treatment of autism, including the Sunderland Protocol, which offers a specific sequence for introducing alternative treatments.

Center for the Study of Autism
c/o Autism Research Institute, 4182 Adams Avenue
San Diego, CA 92116, USA
Website: www.autism.org
This website offers links pertaining to biomedical interventions for autism, including diet and nutrition.

National Institute of Medical Herbalists
56 Longbrook Street
Exeter EX4 AH, UK
Telephone: +44 (0)1392 426 022
Website: www.nimh.org.uk
This is the leading professional organization in the United Kingdom for herbal medical practitioners. It offers training in herbal medicine, and has links for locating qualified practitioners.

ELIMINATION DIETS

Interest in using special diets to manage the behavioral problems in children with neurodevelopmental disorders including autism, ADHD, and other learning differences first gained popularity in the 1970s and early 1980s. Several diets are especially popular and will be discussed here. However, the concept of dietary intervention is very broad, and there are many different theories and types of diets that are being investigated by medical researchers.

Perhaps the most popular current dietary approach is the *gluten-free casein-free (GFCF) diet* used primarily for children with autism spectrum disorders, but sometimes recommended for children with other behavioral problems. Gluten is the protein that is commonly found in wheat, rye, barley, oats, and malt. It is a primary ingredient in most breads and pastas, and is also commonly used as a thickener in soups, gravies, and other prepared foods that contain liquid. Casein is a protein that is found in all products derived from cow's milk. Proponents of the GFCF diet believe that some cases of autism stem from a disorder in the immune system that affects the body's ability to break down these proteins, allowing particles known as *peptides* to remain undigested. These peptides may then cause irritation of the intestinal lining, which results in increased permeability of the lining, popularly referred to as *leaky gut syndrome*. Increased permeability of the intestinal lining allows peptides to flow directly into the bloodstream. These peptides contain high levels of *opioids*, which are similar to heroin and morphine, which can cross the blood-brain barrier and create problems within the nervous system. Children with allergies actually crave the foods that contain these proteins in much the same way as an addict craves drugs. Symptoms of sensitivity to gluten and casein may include vomiting, eczema, ear infections, asthma, and chronic gastrointestinal (GI) problems including diarrhea or constipation. However, proponents warn that some children with sensitivity may be symptom-free. More importantly, proponents of this theory believe that sensitivity to gluten and casein result in cognitive and behavioral changes, and that removing these proteins from the child's diet can, over time, result in improved behavior and cognition.

Implementation of the GFCF diet demands vigilance on the part of parents. Many commercially produced foods contain small amounts of the offending proteins, so parents have to be diligent in knowing exactly what their child consumes on a daily basis, and making sure that the child avoids most convenience foods. Minute amounts of gluten can remain in the body for up to eight months, so parents must commit to a long-term trial of the diet to assure effectiveness. There are manufacturers of GFCF foods, but these tend to be costly and hard to find. As a result, most parents resort to cooking special foods that are GFCF. Some high functioning children are aware of their sensitivity to casein, and self-limit their intake of milk and related products. Gluten, however, tends to create strong cravings, and children are usually resistant to limiting foods that contain this protein. Because of the addictive nature of gluten and casein, the abrupt removal of these proteins from the diet can case severe withdrawal symptoms. Most advocates, therefore, first remove casein from the diet, and then remove gluten at a later time. Research shows conflicting evidence as to the efficacy of this diet; however, there are many parents who claim that it has helped their child.

Children with neurodevelopmental disorders may have other food allergies that can impact their learning and behavior. In children with autism, these sensitivities can be severe. Unfortunately, the type of allergy found in these children does not often show up in routine skin testing for allergies, and can only be determined by systematically eliminating foods that are suspected as being allergens. Problems with bacteria, yeast, or fungus infections affecting the gastrointestinal system may also play a role in how children tolerate different foods, and may require medical interventions, including prescription drugs, to manage these problems. When food intolerance is suspected, parents are encouraged to keep detailed food diaries in an effort to link changes in behavior, sleep patterns, or functional performance to the consumption of specific foods. Foods that are commonly suspected as allergens include eggs, tomatoes, eggplant, avocados, red pepper, soy and corn.

FEINGOLD DIET

Another popular theory of elimination diets stems from the work of allergist Ben Feingold, who introduced the concept of a diet to reduce hyperactivity in children with ADHD in the early 1970s. His theory proposed that many children with attention and learning problems are sensitive to synthetic food colorings, food additives, and salicylates, which are a group of chemicals often included in food additives, but which are also found naturally in such foods as almonds, apples, brazil nuts, broccoli, carrots, grapes, oranges, tomatoes, yeast products, cola, coffee, and tea.

The *Feingold diet* initially restricts all foods that contain synthetic colors, preservatives, or flavors; artificial sweeteners including Aspartame, Neotame, and Alitame; and salicylate-rich foods. Natural foods containing salicylate may be re-introduced one at a time at a later date to determine if any may be tolerated by the child. Contrary to popular tradition, the Feingold diet does not restrict the intake of sugar or chocolate, although moderation is encouraged. Similar to the GFCF diet, the Feingold diet requires parents to be vigilant observers of their child's diet. However, most allowed foods can be easily obtained in regular supermarkets. Some parents choose to reduce, but not fully eliminate, the offensive foods. Strict adherence to this elimination diet is sometimes referred to as the *oligoantigenic diet*. Medical researchers continue to debate the scientific efficacy of the Feingold diet.

Training in elimination diets and the Feingold diet

Many professionals, including doctors, nurses, dieticians, and nutritionists, have training that includes an understanding of the basic nutritional needs of children. Although there are many books and websites that describe the process of implementing an elimination diet, parents are cautioned to do so only after discussing the pros and cons with the child's pediatrician or a qualified nutritionist.

Recommended resources for elimination diets

Literature

Arnold, L.E. (1999) 'Treatment alternatives for attention-deficit/hyperactivity disorders.' *Journal of Attention Disorders, 3*, 1, 30–48.

Christison, G.W. and Ivany, K. (2006) 'Elimination diets in autism spectrum disorders: Any wheat amidst the chaff?' *Journal of Developmental and Behavioral Pediatrics, 27*, 2 suppl., s162–s171.

Elder, J.H., Shankar, M., Shuster, J., Theriaque, D., Burns, S. and Sherrill, L. (2006) 'The gluten-free, casein-free diet in autism: Results of a preliminary double blind clinical trial.' *Journal of Autism and Developmental Disorders, 36*, 3, 413–420.

Horvath, K. and Perman, J.A. (2002) 'Autism and gastrointestinal symptoms.' *Current Gastroenterology Reports, 4*, 3, 251–258.

Jackson, L. and LeBreton, M. (2001) *A User Guide to the GF/CF Diet for Autism, Asperger Syndrome and AD/HD*. London: Jessica Kingsley Publishers.

Le Breton, Marilyn (2001) *Diet Intervention and Autism: Implementing the Gluten Free and Cassein Free Diet for Autistic Children; A Practical Guide for Parents*. London: Jessica Kingsley Publishers.

Lewis, L. and Seroussi, K. (2001) *Special Diets for Special Kids, Two*. Arlington, TX: Future Horizons.

Millward, C., Ferriter, M., Calver, S. and Connell-Jones, G. (2004) 'Gluten-and cassein-free diets for autism spectrum disorder.' *Cochrane Database Systematic Reviews, 2*, CD003498.

Schmidt, M.H., Mocks, P., Lay, B., *et al.* (1997) 'Does oligoantigenic diet influence hyperactive/conduct-disordered children: A controlled trial.' *European Child and Adolescent Psychiatry, 6*, 2, 88–95.

Stevenson, J. (2006) 'Dietary influences on cognitive development and behaviour in children.' *The Proceedings of the Nutrition Society, 65*, 4, 361–365.

Agencies, organizations, and websites

Action Against Allergy
PO Box 278
Twickenham TW1 4QQ, UK
Telephone: +44 (0)208 892 2711
Website: www.actionagainstallergy.co.uk
This agency offers information about diagnosis and treatment of allergies within the National Health System in the United Kingdom.

American Dietetic Association
120 South Riverside Plaza, Suite 2000
Chicago, IL 60606-6995, USA
Telephone: +1 (800) 877-1600
Website: www.eatright.org

Autism Network for Dietary Intervention
PO Box 17711
Rochester, NY 14617-0711, USA
Telephone: +1 (609) 737-8985
Website: www.autismndi.com
This website was established by parent-researchers, and focuses on helping parents of children with autism to understand, implement, and maintain dietary intervention programs. It offers a free newsletter, products, and many helpful articles, some of which have been translated into other languages.

Autism Research Unit (ARU)
School of Health, Natural and Social Sciences
City Campus, University of Sunderland
Sunderland SR1 3SD, UK
Telephone: +44 (0)191 567 0420
Website: http://www.osiris.sunderland.ac.uk/autism
This website offers information about various biomedical interventions for the treatment of autism, including the Sunderland Protocol, which offers a specific sequence for introducing alternative treatments.

British Association of Nutritional Therapists
27 Old Gloucester Road
London WC1N 3XX, UK
Telephone: +44 (0)870 606 1284
Website: www.bant.org.uk

Center for the Study of Autism
c/o Autism Research Institute, 4182 Adams Avenue
San Diego, CA 92116, USA
Website: www.autism.org
This website offers links pertaining to biomedical interventions for autism, including diet and nutrition, including the DAN! protocol.

Feingold Association of the United States
554 East Main Street, Suite 301
Riverhead, NY 11901, USA
Telephone: +1 (800) 321-3287
Website: www.feingold.org

This website offers general information about the Feingold diet, a bookstore, and extensive listings of relevant research. A small membership fee is required to access specific dietary recommendations.

The GFCF Diet Support Group
PO Box 1692
Palm Harbor, FL 34683, USA
Website: www.gfcfdiet.com
This website offers extensive information and products for implementing a gluten-free, casein-free diet.

Hyperactive Children's Support Group (HACSG)
71 Whyke Lane
Chichester, West Sussex PO19 2LD, UK
Telephone: +44 (0)1243 539966 (urgent calls only)
Website: www.hacsg.org.uk

HYPERBARIC OXYGEN THERAPY

Hyperbaric oxygen therapy (HBOT) is a medical treatment that allows oxygen to be quickly absorbed by the brain and other body tissues. This is a treatment that has long been used by scuba divers to treat decompression sickness (the bends), but is also found to increase the amount of oxygen in the cells of the body, which can accomplish several health benefits including: ridding the body of toxins, such as those present in carbon monoxide poisoning; improving blood flow and reducing swelling to tissues that have been infected or injured; and boosting the immune system, which can enhance the ability of white blood cells to fight infection. HBOT is widely used for these medical purposes. More recently, some doctors have claimed that HBOT may be an effective, although controversial, treatment for certain developmental disabilities, including cerebral palsy and autism. The theory behind using HBOT with children who have autism is that the treatment increases oxygen to brain tissues, helping to stimulate neurological function and possibly to regenerate damaged brain tissue. It is also used in conjunction with chelation therapy and other treatments designed to detoxify the body from heavy metals such as mercury.

The procedure involves having the child sit or lie in a pressurized chamber while breathing oxygen-enriched air or pure oxygen. The amount of pressure and oxygen needed are determined by the doctor and the particular protocol he or she is following. Many different kinds of chambers may be used, depending on the service provider. Traditional chambers are large enough for more than one person to sit inside. The pressure is gradually increased while the child is inside the chamber, and the child breathes the enriched air through a helmet placed over the head, or through a flexible mask placed over the nose or mouth. These larger chambers allow a parent to accompany the child, and it is possible to read, watch television, or listen to music during the procedure which typically lasts for an hour or more. Some facilities use smaller chambers that are only large enough to accommodate the child. These smaller chambers are flooded with the air, so the child does not have to wear a helmet or mask. For the treatment of children with autism some doctors recommend portable HBOT chambers which can be used for home treatment. These are usually called *mild chambers*, because they provide less atmospheric pressure than the larger chambers. Protocols vary from child to child, but typically involve several treatments per week for several weeks.

HBOT is generally a painless procedure, but some children experience popping in their ears, sinus pressure, dental pain, or temporary vision changes. There are some more serious potential risks, including the possibility of oxygen toxicity which could cause seizures. For this reason, the treatment must be closely supervised by a qualified physician.

Because HBOT has not been scientifically proven to be an effective treatment for children with developmental disabilities including autism, it is often not reimbursed by insurance, and can be an extremely costly undertaking for those parents who must pay the full cost of the procedure. As a treatment, it is more widely available in the United Kingdom than in the United States, where there is a shortage of facilities and doctors trained in the procedure.

Training in hyperbaric oxygen therapy

This is a medical intervention that must be prescribed by and supervised by qualified doctors. Doctors who are trained in European schools of medicine often receive more exposure to this intervention than doctors who train in the United States, and may therefore be more familiar with the procedure. In the United Kingdom, this therapy may be financed through the National Health Service or through some non-profit medical centers. In the United States, the intervention is approved by Medicare and the FDA for certain conditions such as severe wounds or carbon monoxide poisoning, but is generally not approved for use in treating developmental disabilities where its effectiveness has not been satisfactorily established through controlled double-blind studies.

Recommended resources for hyperbaric oxygen therapy

Literature

Golden, Z., Golden, C.J. and Neubauer, R.A. (2006) 'Improving neuropsychological function after chronic brain injury with hyperbaric oxygen.' *Disability and Rehabilitation, 28,* 22, 1379–1386.

Golden, Z.L., Neubauer, R., Golden, C.J., Greene, L, Marsh, J. and Mieko, A. (2002) 'Improvement in cerebral metabolism in chronic brain injury after hyperbaric oxygen therapy.' *The International Journal of Neuroscience, 112,* 2, 119–131.

Harch, P.G. and McCullough, V. (2007) *The Oxygen Revolution: Hyperbaric Oxygen Therapy: The Groundbreaking New Treatment for Stroke, Alzheimer's, Parkinson's, Arthritis, Autism, Learning Disabilities and More.* Long Island City, NY: Hatherleigh Press.

Rossignol, D.A. (2006) 'Hyperbaric oxygen therapy might improve certain pathophysiological findings in autism.' *Medical Hypotheses, 68,* 6, 1208–1227.

Stoller, K.P. (2005) 'Quantification of neurocognitive changes before, during, and after hyperbaric oxygen therapy in a case of fetal alcohol syndrome.' *Pediatrics, 116,* 4, 586–591.

Agencies, organizations, and websites

HBOTreatment.com
e-mail: info@HBOTreatment.com
Telephone: +1 (770) 246-4469
This is an educational website offering information about the uses of hyperbaric oxygen therapy for various conditions.

International Hyperbarics Association, Inc.
15810 East Gale Avenue #178
Hacienda Heights, CA 91746, USA
Telephone: +1 (877) 442-8721
Website: www.ihausa.org
This is an educational and charitable organization focusing on the needs of the hyperbaric community. It distributes and publishes data, articles, and papers; supports research; offers grants to those in need of hyperbaric oxygen therapy. It also provides information on where to access the treatment in the United States.

IMMUNE SYSTEM THERAPY (IGG, IVIG)

Some children with autism present with certain immunological abnormalities which suggest the possibility that autoimmune problems may be causing or contributing to the symptoms of autism. Because of this, there is growing interest in the possible use of *intravenous immunoglobulin treatment (IVIG)* to improve autistic symptoms. *Immunoglobulins* are proteins that are naturally manufactured by the body. They produce antibodies that serve to communicate with immune system cells and modify the immune reaction. Immunoglobulin products were first used in the early 1950s to treat patients with leukemia and immune deficiency. Since the 1950s, IVIG therapy has been successfully used to treat a wide variety of autoimmune disorders. The FDA in the United States approves the use of IVIG for a number of conditions, for example primary immunodeficiency, Kawasaki disease, certain types of leukemia, pediatric HIV infection, and prevention of graft versus host disease in transplant patients, to list a few. It is not approved at this time for treatment of autism but is being used in a number of clinical trials to determine its potential impact on children with this diagnosis. Treatment is usually conducted on an outpatient basis, and involves a series of intravenous injections. This is an extremely costly procedure, more so in the United States than in the United Kingdom, and also has the potential to cause adverse effects. Studies suggest that adverse effects may be seen in 1 percent to 15 percent of patients, depending on the particular product used. Products that use sugars, especially sucrose, seem to be particularly prone to causing adverse effects. Some adverse effects are mild, including redness, eczema, or swelling at the injection site; headaches or backaches; nausea and vomiting; chills and fever; hypotension or hypertension; and rashes. However, there is some potential for serious and even fatal side effects resulting from aseptic meningitis, renal failure, or vascular thrombosis.

Training in immune system therapy

Immune system therapy is a medical procedure that has the potential for serious adverse effects. It is a specialized treatment that is considered experimental and unproven when used for children with autism, and at this time must be provided by a qualified physician as part of a formal research protocol.

Recommended resources for immune system therapy

Literature

Kazatchkine, M.D. (ed.) (1995) *Intravenous Immunoglobulin Therapy – Clinical Benefits and Future Prospects.* New York: The Parthenon Publishing Group.

Ploplys, A.V. (1998) 'Intravenous immunoglobulin treatment of children with autism.' *Journal of Child Neurology, 13.* 2, 79–82.

Ploplys, A.V. (2000) 'Intravenous immunoglobulin treatment in autism.' *Journal of Autism and Developmental Disorders, 30,* 1, 73–74.

Wiles, C.M., Brown, P., Chapel, H., *et al.* (2002) 'Intravenous immunoglobulin in neurological disease: A specialist review.' *Journal of Neurology, Neurosurgery and Psychiatry, 72*, 440–448.

Agencies, organizations, and websites

Autism Independent UK
(Formerly Society for the Autistically Handicapped–SFTAH)
199–203 Blandford Avenue
Kettering, Northants NN16 9AT, UK
Telephone: +44 (0)1536 523274
Website: www.autismuk.com
This society serves to increase awareness of autism by providing information, resources and training to professionals and non-professionals. Among other extensive resources, it has a section that lists a comprehensive review of available research pertaining to IVIG therapy for children with autism.

Chapter 6

MANIPULATIVE
AND BODY-BASED METHODS

ALEXANDER TECHNIQUE

The *Alexander technique* is an educational program that strives to teach students how to change poor posture and movement patterns with the goal of improving coordination and balance, reducing tension and fatigue, improving certain medical conditions, and promoting general well-being. This intervention is named for Matthias Alexander, a Shakespearean actor who developed the technique between 1890 and 1900 to correct his own problems with his voice and acting performance. Alexander observed that when he assumed certain constricted postures of his back and neck, he lost his voice, but when he corrected his posture, his voice returned. He postulated that all children are born with freedom of movement, but as they gradually adjust to the stresses of everyday life, they draw their bodies into defensive postures that restrict their freedom of movement. A major premise of the intervention is that all people create habits as they react to circumstances, because habits help behavior to become more simplified. However, movement habits can be harmful, as repetition decreases the person's sense of the movement (*proprioception*), so they become less and less aware of the effectiveness of their movement. Teachers of the Alexander technique guide students to learn proper movement habits and to increase their sensory awareness of movement through verbal direction and light touch, usually requiring as many as 20 to 40 sessions to teach the student to learn the technique. Most widely used by actors, singers, and athletes, the technique is also used for patients with autism and learning disabilities who have problems with coordination. Because the patient needs to cognitively learn the importance of the technique, it may be more applicable to older children and adults, although some proponents believe it can be helpful for children as young as six years.

Training in the Alexander technique

Certification in teaching the Alexander technique is available to students who have completed at least three years of undergraduate study and have themselves received instruction in the Alexander technique. The certification process generally involves 1600 hours of training over a three-year period of time in an approved program.

Recommended resources for the Alexander technique

Literature

Gelb, M.J. (1996) *Body Learning: An Introduction to the Alexander Technique.* New York: Owl Books.

Jain, S., Janssen, K. and DeCelle, S. (2004) 'Alexander technique and Feldenkrais method: A critical overview.' *Physical Medicine and Rehabilitation Clinics of North America, 15,* 4, 811–825.

Maitland, S. (1996) 'An exploration of the application of the Alexander technique for people with learning disabilities.' *British Journal of Learning Disabilities, 24,* 70–76.

Nuttall, W. (1999) 'The Alexander principle: A consideration of its relevance to early childhood education in England today.' *European Early Childhood Education Research Journal, 7,* 2, 87–101.

Vineyard, M. (2007) *How You Stand, How You Move, How You Live: Learning the Alexander Technique to Explore Your Mind-Body Connection and Achieve Self-Mastery.* New York: Marlowe and Company.

Agencies, organizations, and websites

Alexander Technique Worldwide
Website: www.alexandertechniqueworldwide.com
This is an international organization that provides a directory of professional societies involved with the Alexander Technique worldwide.

American Society for the Alexander Technique
PO Box 60008
Florence, MA 01062, USA
Telephone: +1 (800) 473-0620
Website: www.alexandertech.com

Society of Teachers for the Alexander Technique (STAT)
1st Floor, Linton House, 39–51 Highgate Road
London NW5 1RS, UK
Telephone: +44 (0)845 230 7828
Website: www.stat.org.uk

BRAIN GYM®

Brain Gym®, one aspect of a therapeutic intervention approach known as *Educational Kinesiology (EDU-K)*, is a system of physical movement exercises designed to help children and adults to overcome learning and behavioral problems through exercise. It is based upon the premise that successful brain function requires efficient connections across the neural pathways located in the brain, and that stress can inhibit these connections. Specially designed exercises are thought to stimulate a flow of information across these connections, restoring the innate ability to learn. The methodology was first developed in the 1970s by an American educational specialist, Paul Dennison, along with his wife, Gail E. Dennison, and is now widely used across the world in schools, athletic training programs, performing arts programs, and in some corporate programs. The Brain Gym® program includes 26 exercises organized around three dimensions. *Laterality* involves exercises that require the person to physically cross the midline of the body so that both hemispheres of the brain are working simultaneously. This is believed to be an important neurological function of reading, writing, and communicating. *Focus* exercises are designed to coordinate the front and back portions of the brain, a process believed to improve comprehension and the ability to use and express information stored in the brain, as needed for speaking, test taking, or creative expression. *Centering* exercises help coordinate the top and bottom areas of the brain, which is believed to increase the flow of energy moving through the body, helping to release stress and fatigue, and to make one feel more grounded and ready for learning. Brain Gym® exercises can be used by teachers and parents with minimal instruction as part of a daily routine, or may be individually prescribed by a licensed Brain Gym® instructor. The exercises are quick and fun for children, with interesting names like "brain buttons" or "double doodles".

Training in Brain Gym®

Professionals from a variety of backgrounds can become licensed as a Brain Gym® Instructor/Consultant through a combination of courses, consultations, and case studies approved through the Educational Kinesiology Foundation. The foundation also offers a variety of workshops and inservices to agencies and organizations worldwide. A number of books and publications are available that describe how parents and teachers can incorporate exercises into the daily routines of children.

Recommended resources for Brain Gym®

Literature

Cohen, I. and Goldsmith, M. (2002) *Hands On: How to Use Brain Gym® in the Classroom.* Ventura, CA: Edu-Kinesthetics, Inc.

Dennison, P.E. and Dennison, G.E. (1992) *Brain Gym®: Simple Activities for Whole Brain Learning.* Ventura, CA: Edu-Kinesthetics, Inc.

Khalsa, G.C.K., Morris, D. and Sifft, J.M. (1988) 'The effects of Educational Kinesiology on the static balance of learning-disabled students.' *Perceptual and Motor Skills, 67*, 51–54.

Agencies, organizations, and websites

The Educational Kinesiology Foundation/Brain Gym® International
1575 Spinnaker Drive, Suite 204B
Ventura, CA 93001, USA
Telephone: +1 (800) 356-2109
Website: www.braingym.org
This is the official website of the Educational Kinesiology Foundation, offering information about Brain Gym® methods, training opportunities, publications, and links to worldwide distributors of books and products, and an international listing of licensed practitioners.

Educational Kinesiology UK Foundation
12, Golders Rise
London NW4 2HR, UK
Telephone: +44 (0)208 202 3141
Website: www.braingym.org.uk
The official organization for Brain Gym® in the United Kingdom and Europe.

CHIROPRACTIC

Chiropractic is a complementary and alternative profession that is focused on improving health and nervous system functioning through manipulations of the joints and vertebrae. Chiropractors believe that misalignment of the spine, pelvis, or skull (called *subluxations*) causes pinching (*entrapment*) of nerves that are protected by the spinal column, potentially leading to a variety of health problems, including pain. Because the central nervous system serves to regulate all bodily functions, the release of these subluxations is believed to have effects that can go far beyond the relief of pain. For example, subluxations around the cranial areas of the spine are believed to cause interruption to efficient functioning of the cranial nerves, and may lead to some of the eye-hand coordination and perceptual difficulties common among children with learning disabilities or autism.

Chiropractic treatment involves a variety of spinal manipulations (called *adjustments*) that attempt to release restrictions in the spine. Most chiropractors limit their treatment approach to these adjustments, and refer to themselves as *straights*. Others combine adjustments with other *naturopathic* interventions, such as diet and exercise, and consider themselves to be primary health care providers. Those who use other modalities in addition to manipulation are called *mixers*.

Although generally considered a safe intervention, chiropractic is not recommended for patients with certain health conditions, including spinal tumors or inflammation, recent bone fractures, or osteoporosis. On rare occasions, serious adverse effects, including hemorrhage or paralysis, have been reported. Some critics express concern that the use of full spine X-rays to detect subluxations are necessary and could expose the patient to radiation risk. They also fear that certain treatable medical conditions may not be recognized by mixed chiropractors, and may therefore not receive early diagnosis and treatment.

Training in chiropractic

In the United States, students must successfully complete a four-year program leading to a degree of Doctor of Chiropractic (DC). To become licensed, they must pass examinations given by the National Board of Chiropractic Examiners, and must meet other state-specific requirements, which may include other undergraduate preparation. Chiropractic colleges also offer post-doctoral training in several areas, including pediatrics, which leads to "diplomate" status in the specialty area.

In the United Kingdom, students must graduate from a college approved by the General Chiropractic Council (GCC) with either a Bachelor of science or undergraduate Master's degree, and must register with the GCC in order to practice.

Recommended resources for chiropractic

Literature

Breunner, C. (2002) 'Complementary medicine in pediatrics: A review of acupuncture, homeopathy, massage, and chiropractic therapies.' *Current Problems in Pediatric and Adolescent Health Care, 32*, 10, 353–384.

Giesen, J.M., Center, D.B. and Leach, R.A. (1989) 'An evaluation of chiropractic manipulation as a treatment of hyperactivity in children.' *Journal of Manipulative and Physiological Therapeutics, 12*, 5, 353–363.

Jennings, J. and Barker, M. (2006) 'Autism: A chiropractic perspective.' *Clinical Chiropractic, 9*, 1, 6–10.

Meeker, W.C. and Haldeman, S. (2002) 'Chiropractic: A profession at the crossroads of mainstream and alternative medicine.' *Annals of Internal Medicine, 136*, 3, 216–227.

Mootz, R.D. and Bowers, L.J. (eds.) (1999) *Chiropractic Care of Special Populations (Topics in Clinical Chiropractic Series)*. Sudbury, MA: Jones and Bartlett Publishers.

Vohra, S., Johnston, B.C., Cramer, K. and Humphreys, K. (2007) 'Adverse effects associated with pediatric spinal manipulation: A systematic review.' *Pediatrics, 119*, 1, 275–283.

Yannick, P. (2007) 'The effects of chiropractic care on individuals suffering from learning disabilities and dyslexia: A review of the literature.' *Journal of Vertebral Subluxation Research*, January 15, 1–12.

Agencies, organizations, and websites

American Chiropractic Association
1701 Clarendon Boulevard
Arlington, VA 22209, USA
Telephone: +1 (703) 276-8800
Website: www.acatoday.com
This is the largest organization in the world representing doctors of chiropractic.

British Chiropractic Association
59 Castle Street
Reading, Berkshire RG1 7SN, UK
Telephone: +44 (0)1189 505950
Website: www.chiropractic-uk.co.uk
This is the largest member organization for chiropractors in the United Kingdom.

General Chiropractic Council
44 Wicklow Street
London WC1X 9HL, UK
Telephone: +44 (0)207 713 5155
Website: www.gcc-uk.org
This is a statutory body that sets standards for education and registers qualified chiropractors in the United Kingdom. It offers publications, links to related websites, and a locator service for consumers.

National Board of Chiropractic Examiners
901 54th Avenue
Greely, CO 80634, USA
Telephone: +1 (970) 356-9100
Website: www.nbce.org
This is a non-profit national and international testing organization for the
chiropractic profession, offering examinations to students in the United States,
Canada, France, and Australia.

CONDUCTIVE EDUCATION

Conductive education is a system of education designed for children and adults with
problems affecting motor control and coordination. Originally designed for
patients with cerebral palsy or other serious neurologically based motor disabilities, it also has application for children and adults with milder forms of motor
disabilities, including dyspraxia. This system of education was pioneered by a
Hungarian doctor, Andras Petö, in the 1940s, and is now used worldwide, especially for children with cerebral palsy. Proponents of conductive education
believe that the child is able and wants to learn, even in the presence of damage
to the central nervous system, through a cognitive approach to teaching and
learning. Methods are based upon the theory that the central nervous system has
the ability to form new neurological connections leading to desired movements
despite injury to the nervous system. Rather than a specific set of exercises or
techniques, it is a complete educational system that is intended to promote a
"way of life" throughout the child's day. The method involves having the child
perform a range of daily living tasks, ranging from feeding and dressing to basic
mobility skills, while a trained *conductor* motivates the child to identify and
achieve his or her personal goals. The intervention requires many hours per day
of intervention, with extensive parent training and involvement. The most
important functions of the conductor include: encouraging consistent and
strong motivation to learn to perform daily life skills despite the disability; stimulating activity and ability through interesting, playful, and emotionally engaging
activities; and supporting the child in finding solutions to fulfill all cultural and
social requirements within the mainstream setting. The program often incorporates the use of specialized furniture, including plinths, ladders, and slatted
chairs, to entice children to reach out, stabilize themselves, and become active
within their environment. Of greatest importance is the strength of the
personal relationship between the conductor and the child. When successful,
the end result is that the child learns to become independent in life tasks by com-
pensating for neurological injury.

Training in conductive education

Conductive education is primarily taught at the Petö Institute in Budapest, Hungary, and requires six years of course and practicum training, and passing a national examination to achieve certification. The Petö Institute directs and supervises other training centers throughout the world.

Recommended resources for conductive education

Literature

Kozma, I. and Balogh, E. (1975) 'A brief introduction to conductive education and its application at an early age.' *Infants and Young Children, 8*, 1, 68–74.

Kozma, I. (1995) 'The basic principles and the present practice of conductive education.' *European Journal of Special Needs Education, 10*, 2, 111–123.

Rózsahegyi, T. (2003) 'Conductive education: A different kind of training.' *Primary Practice*, (84): 45–48.

Russell, A. (1994) *Evaluation of Conductive Education: A Statistical Overkill Challenging the Scientific Validity and Harsh Conclusion of a University of Birmingham Trial.* London: Acorn Foundation Publications.

Spivack, F. (1995) 'Conductive education perspectives.' *Infants and Young Children, 8*, 1, 75–85.

Tatlow, A. (2006) 'Conductive education for children with cerebral palsy. Hong Kong Spastic Association.' *Recent Advances in Conductive Education, 6*, 1, 33–34.

Agencies, organizations, and websites

Conductive Learning Center
2428 Burton Street S.E.
Grand Rapids, MI 4954, USA
Telephone: +1 (616) 575-0575
Website: www.aquinas.edu/clc
Located at Aquinas College, this center offers conductive education programs for children from infancy through adolescence. It is the only program in North America that is directed and supervised by the International Petö Institute of Conductive Education in Budapest, Hungary, and offers a conductor-teacher preparation program.

Inter-American Conductive Education Association
PO Box 3169
Toms River, NJ 08756-3169, USA
Telephone:+1 (800) 824-2332 (toll-free from within United States)
          +1 (732) 797-2566
Website: www.iacea.org

This organization is devoted to promoting resources and awareness of conductive education in North America, including links to agencies providing conductive education services.

International Petö Institute of Conductive Education
Website: www.peto.hu

The Foundation for Conductive Education
Canon Hill House, Russell Road
Birmingham B13 8RD, UK
Telephone: +44 (0)121 449 1569
Website: www.conductive-education.org.uk
This organization serves as a center of excellence for the development of conductive education in the United Kingdom, offering direct services, professional training, and an extensive collection of literature focusing on research and development.

CRANIOSACRAL THERAPY

Craniosacral therapy (sometimes referred to as *cranial osteopathy*) is a manual therapy that involves gentle manipulation of the cranial bones and spine in the belief that this will improve the function of the central nervous system. It is usually performed by osteopathic physicians, chiropractors, physical therapists, occupational therapists, massage therapists, or others who have professional training in human anatomy and function. The theory behind this approach is based on several key points. We know that the central nervous system (including the brain and spinal column) is surrounded by a fluid (*cerebrospinal fluid*, or *CSF*) that flows continuously throughout the system. A serious blockage of the flow of this fluid causes the fluid to accumulate in the brain, causing the condition known as *hydrocephalus*. Craniosacral therapists believe that there are much more subtle anatomical conditions that slightly disrupt the normal flow of CSF, causing disease, stress, or pain. These disruptions may be caused by slight misalignment of the bones of the skull along their sutures, by stress and tension within the body, or by traumatic injury. Craniosacral therapists further believe that the human brain has rhythmic movements, unrelated to heart rate or breathing, that can be detected by placing the fingertips gently on the skull. Aberrant rhythms are believed to indicate disease. Unfortunately, research has shown that there is poor reliability of these measurements, even among trained craniosacral therapists.

Proponents of craniosacral therapy suggest that it may be an alternative medical intervention for children with a wide range of disorders, including developmental delay, autism, ADHD, learning disabilities, strabismus, brain injuries, and orthopedic problems such as torticollis. The method involves applying extremely light touch (less than 5 grams) on various parts of the skull and body while the child remains fully clothed. Sessions may last from 15 to 60 minutes, depending on the child's tolerance to remaining still. While touching the child, the therapist is attempting to interpret the rhythm of CSF flowing through the body, while gently releasing restrictions that may be caused by bony or tissue tightness. It is considered a safe intervention, with very few concerns about possible side effects.

Training in craniosacral therapy

Craniosacral therapy is not formally regulated in either the United States or the United Kingdom. In the United States, the Upledger Institute offers a voluntary certification program that includes four levels of training. Acceptance into this training is limited to students who have some prior background in anatomy and health care. Voluntary certification is also offered through the Craniosacral Association of North America, which requires three years of training. In the United Kingdom, voluntary registration is offered through the Cranio Sacral Society, which adheres to the Upledger method, and through the Craniosacral Therapy Association of the UK. Most craniosacral therapists are regulated through their professional training as osteopaths, occupational or physical therapists, chiropractors, or massage therapists.

Recommended resources for craniosacral therapy

Literature

Cohen, D. and Upledger, J.E. (1996) *An Introduction to Craniosacral Therapy: Anatomy, Function, and Treatment.* Berkeley, CA: North Atlantic Books.

Downey, P.A., Barbano, T., Kapur-Wadhwa, R., Sciote, J.J., Siegel, M.I. and Mooney, M.P. (2006) 'Craniosacral therapy: The effects of cranial manipulation on intracranial pressure and cranial bone movement.' *Journal of Orthopedic and Sports Physical Medicine, 36*, 11, 845–853.

Green, C., Martin, C.W., Bassett, K. and Kazanjian, A. (1999) 'A systematic review of craniosacral therapy: Biological plausibility, assessment reliability, and clinical effectiveness.' *Complementary Therapies in Medicine, 7*, 4, 201–207.

Upledger, J.E. (1997) *A Brain is Born: Exploring the Birth and Development of the Central Nervous System.* Berkeley, CA: North Atlantic Books.

Wirth-Patulo, V. and Hayes, K.W. (1994) 'Interrater reliability of craniosacral rate measurements and their relationship with subjects' and examiners' heart and respiratory rate measurements.' *Physical Therapy, 74*, 10, 908–916.

Agencies, organizations, and websites

Biodynamic Craniosacral Therapy Association of North America
852 Don Diego Avenue
Santa Fe, NM 87505, USA
Telephone: +1 (505) 820-1355
Website: www.craniosacraltherapy.org
This organization was founded to establish curriculum, approve teachers, and register therapists. It also provides a referral service to consumers interested in finding a registered craniosacral therapist.

The Upledger Institute, Inc.
11211 Prosperity Farms Road, Suite D-325
Palm Beach Gardens, FL 33410, USA
Telephone: +1 (561) 622-4334
Website: www.upledger.com
This is the website of John Upledger, DO, who is the foremost proponent of craniosacral therapy. The site offers extensive information, training opportunities, and links to other sites.

The Cranio Sacral Society
2 Marshall Place
Perth PH2 8AH, Scotland
Telephone: +44 (0)1738 444404
Website: www.cranio-sacral.org.uk
This is the practitioner organization for Upledger craniosacral therapy in the United Kingdom. It offers training leading to voluntary registration, as well as help with finding local practitioners.

The Craniosacral Therapy Association of the United Kingdom
Monomark House, 27 Old Gloucester Street
London WC1N 3XX, UK
Telephone: +44 (0)7000 784 735
Website: www.craniosacral.co.uk
This organization offers voluntary registration to practitioners who successfully graduate from an accredited training school or college.

DEVELOPMENTAL/BEHAVIORAL OPTOMETRY

Screening for vision problems is part of routine pediatric health care, and is effective in identifying problems with eye health, structure, or significant vision impairment. However, milder problems with vision may go undetected during routine vision screenings. Difficulty with using vision efficiently, also called *functional vision impairment*, and problems with interpreting or understanding what is seen, called *visual perception disorders* are common in autism and in some types of learning disability, especially non-verbal learning disability. There also appears to be a link between ADHD and certain types of visual perception difficulty. *Developmental/behavioral optometry* addresses these concerns. In addition to providing basic eyecare, a developmental/behavioral optometrist offers a more holistic approach to the treatment of vision disorders, and is focused on the role that vision plays in the child's daily activities. They provide a more comprehensive assessment of how efficiently vision is used for learning and everyday functioning, and provide specialized intervention for problems with lazy eyes, poor eye teaming and tracking, visual motor integration problems, and visual perceptual disorders. Intervention, often referred to as *vision therapy,* may include special lenses, eye exercises, and other training methods designed to strengthen the eyes and reduce visual stress so that vision may be used more efficiently. They also provide consultation to parents and school personnel regarding accommodations that may help to reduce visual stress. Although vision therapy is considered controversial in mainstream medicine, there is growing documentation of research supporting its use.

Training in developmental/behavioral optometry

Optometrists must complete a four year graduate program in optometry, and use the initials OD after their name. General optometrists may provide vision therapy as part of their practice, but post-graduate training is available to those who choose to specialize in working with children. In the United States, two organizations offer examinations for optometrists to assess their level of expertise in this area. Those who pass the examination given by the American Academy of Optometry are called Diplomates in Binocular Vision, Perception, and Pediatric Optometry. Those who pass the examination offered by the College of Optometrists in Vision Development (COVD) are called Fellows of the COVD, and use the initials FCOVD after their name. Either of these advanced credentials assures extensive post-graduate study. Behavioral optometrists in the United Kingdom are accredited and regulated by the British Association of Behavioral Optometrists.

Recommended resources for developmental/behavioral optometry

Literature

Bowen, M.D. (2002) 'Learning disabilities, dyslexia, and vision: A subject review.' *Optometry, 73,* 553–575.

Cooper, J. (1998) 'Summary of research on the efficacy of vision therapy for specific visual dysfunctions.' *The Journal of Behavioral Optometry*, *9*, 5, 115–119.

Cuiffreda, K.J. (2002) 'The scientific basis for and efficacy of optometric vision therapy in nonstrabismic accommodative and vergence disorders.' *Optometry*, *73*, 735–762.

Hurst, C.M., Van de Weyer, S., Smith, C. and Adler, P.M. (2006) 'Improvements in performance following optometric vision therapy in a child with dyspraxia.' *Ophthalmic and Physiological Optics: The Journal of the British College of Ophthalmic Opticians*, *26*, 2, 199–210.

Kaplan, M. (2005) *Seeing Through New Eyes: Changing the Lives of Autistic Children, Asperger Syndrome, and Other Developmental Disabilities Through Vision Therapy.* London: Jessica Kingsley Publishers.

Kurtz, L.A. (2006) *Visual Perception Problems in Children with AD/HD, Autism, and Other Learning Disabilities: A Guide for Parents and Professionals.* London: Jessica Kingsley Publishers.

Maples, W.C. (2003) 'Visual factors that significantly impact academic performance.' *Optometry*, *4*, 35–49.

Scheiman, M., Mitchell, G.L., Cotter, S., *et al.* The Convergence Insufficiency Treatment Trial Study Group (2005) 'A randomized clinical trial of treatments for convergence insufficiency in children.' *Archives of Ophthalmology*, *123*, 1, 14–24.

Agencies, organizations, and websites

All About Vision Consumer Guide

Website: www.allaboutvision.com

This website offers an extensive consumer guide on subjects relating to eye health, vision care, and learning disabilities.

American Academy of Optometry

6110 Executive Boulevard, Suite 506
Rockville, MD 20852, USA
Telephone: +1 (301) 984-1441
Website: www.aaopt.org

American Academy of Optometry (British Chapter)

2 Doric Place
Woodbridge, Suffolk IP12 1BT, UK
Telephone: +44 (0)1394 380139
Website: www.academy.org.uk

British Association of Behavioral Optometrists
Website: www.babo.co.uk
This website offers an on-line listing of behavioral optometrists who practice throughout the UK.

College of Optometrists in Vision Development
215 West Garfield Road, Suite 210
Aurora, OH 44202, USA
Telephone: +1 (330) 995-0718
Website: www.covd.org
This organization offers extensive resources for parents and professionals, along with a directory of qualified professionals. It has useful articles about the role of vision in autism, ADHD, and learning disabilities.

Optometric Extension Program
1921 E. Carnegie Avenue, Suite 3-L
Santa Ana, CA 92705-5510, USA
Telephone: +1 (949) 250-8070
Website: www.oep.org
This website provides extensive articles and resources for parents and professionals, along with an on-line store for books relating to vision and disabilities.

FELDENKRAIS

The *Feldenkrais* method is an educational system that uses movement and self-awareness activities to reduce pain or restrictions in movement, to improve coordination, or to promote overall well-being and personal development. It is commonly used to treat chronic pain or neuromuscular conditions such as cerebral palsy, and to improve self-awareness in dancers and other performers. It is also proposed as a useful method for improving balance and coordination problems that may occur in children with learning disabilities. This method was developed by Moshé Feldenkrais, who was an Israeli physicist, scientist, engineer, and accomplished judo practitioner. It became popular during the 1970s, and the tradition has been carried on by a small number of practitioners who personally trained under Dr Feldenkrais. Rather than attempting to diagnose or treat illness or disability, the Feldenkrais method is a holistic approach to help people become more aware of how they move. Instructors do not consider the method to be a form of therapy, but an exercise in self-awareness. Feldenkrais believed that this unique method of mind/body exploration ultimately leads to improved health and emotional maturity.

There are two levels of Feldenkrais intervention. *Awareness Through Movement* involves an instructor who verbally directs students to perform slow, non-aerobic movement sequences, and to become more aware of how specific movements contribute to function. With children, these exercises often take the form of creative play, such as wearing masks while imitating the movements of various animals to music. *Functional Integration* is a hands-on form of the Feldenkrais method, that involves the instructor gently manipulating joints and muscles to help patients think about and change their movement habits. All movements are done at a pace that is comfortable for the student, are guided but not forced by the instructor, and are designed to help the student move with less effort and with more freedom of movement. In applying the method, great emphasis is placed on the relationship between the instructor and the student. Proponents believe that change occurs not through simply asking the student to move, or guiding the movement, but in becoming one with the patient. The instructor must learn to interact with the student so the two become a single system, sometimes thought of as a "dance" between the instructor and the student. Instructors usually work with students for four to six sessions which may be repeated periodically over time. Students can practice the techniques at home once they have mastered basic understanding of the method.

Although there are many anecdotal claims of improvements in self-awareness, pain reduction, and improved motor skills, there is limited scientific evidence to support these claims. Critics claim that although there are many published studies, most are flawed due to methodological weaknesses.

Training in the Feldenkrais method

Providers of the Feldenkrais method may include lay practitioners, as well as those with other professional backgrounds such as physical or occupational therapists. The practice is not formally regulated in either the United States or the United Kingdom. Several organizations oversee the accreditation of training programs in the Feldenkrais method and set standards for education and practice. Generally, training requires approximately 800 hours of instruction conducted over a period of four years. After two years, trainees are considered certified to teach Awareness Through Movement to the public. Trainees who complete the full four-year program are eligible to become members of the Feldenkrais Guild, and can teach both Awareness Through Movement and Functional Integration.

Recommended resources for the Feldenkrais method

Literature

Buchanan, P.A. and Ulrich, B.D. (2001) 'The Feldenkrais Method: A dynamic approach to changing motor behavior.' *Research Quarterly for Exercise and Sport, 74*, 2, 124–126.

Feldenkrais, M. (1991) *Awareness Through Movement: Easy-to-Do Health Exercises to Improve Your Posture, Vision, Imagination, and Personal Awareness.* San Francisco, CA: Harper.

Feldenkrais, M. (2002) *The Potent Self: A Study of Spontaneity and Compulsion.* Berkeley, CA: North Atlantic Books/Frog Ltd.

Ives, J.C. and Shelley, G.A. (1998) 'The Feldenkrais Method in rehabilitation: A review.' *WORK: A Journal of Prevention, Assessment and Rehabilitation, 11*, 75–80.

Jain, S., Janssen, K. and DeCelle, S. (2004) 'Alexander technique and Feldenkrais method: A critical overview.' *Physical Medicine and Rehabilitation Clinics of North America, 15*, 4, 811–825.

Rosenholtz, S. (1991) *Move Like the Animals.* New York: Lothrop, Lee and Shepard Books.

Agencies, organizations, and websites

European Training Accreditation Board
c/o Feldenkrais-Gilde Deutschland e.V.
Jaegerwirtstr. 3, D-81373, Munich, Germany
Telephone: +49 (0)89 72 62 55 90
Website: www.eurotab.org
This organization offers accreditation and oversight of Feldenkrais Method training programs in Europe.

Feldenkrais Guild of North America
5436 N. Albina Avenue
Portland, OR 97239, USA
Telephone: +1 (503) 221-6612
Website: www.feldenkrais.com
This organization offers access to research articles, and on-line bookstore, and referrals to trained practitioners in the United States and Canada.

Feldenkrais Guild UK
c/o Scott Clark
13 Camelia House
Idonia Street, London SE8 4LZ, UK
Telephone: +44 (0)7000 785 506
Website: www.feldenkrais.co.uk

This is a professional organization that offers directories of classes, workshops, and trained practitioners in the United Kingdom.

Feldenkrais Resources
830 Bancroft Way, Suite 112
Berkeley, CA 94701, USA
Telephone: +1 (800) 765-1907
Website: www.feldenkrais-resources.com
This website is a clearinghouse for books, materials, and other products relating to the Feldenkrais Method.

International Feldenkrais Federation
Website: www.feldenkrais-method.org
This is the official agency for developing international standards of practice in the Feldenkrais Method. It includes a bibliography of references as well as links to member organizations throughout the world.

HIGASHI (DAILY LIFE THERAPY)

Higashi, also called *Daily Life Therapy*, is a unique educational methodology that was developed by a Japanese educator, Kiyo Kitahara, in the early 1960s. Rather than a specific technique, Higashi is a holistic approach to educating children with autism. Its main focus is to provide gentle, systematic guidance to help students develop confidence and self-esteem through gaining independence in daily living skills. Behavior is managed by emphasizing the student's strengths, providing positive role models, and giving consistent verbal and physical prompts to discourage undesired behaviors. Dr Kitahara believed that medication for managing behavior is incompatible with Daily Life Therapy because of its potential side effects, and because it interferes with the student's ability to learn to self-regulate. Therefore, students enrolled in her program are not permitted to take medication for behavioral or emotional concerns.

The second focus of the method is the use of extensive physical exercise as a connection to social development. Students participate in daily, rigorous exercise and physically active play. This is believed to reduce anxiety through the release of natural neurotransmitters called *endorphins*, and helps reduce aggression, self-stimulatory behaviors, and wakefulness at night. Also, as students gain control over their bodies, they learn to cooperate and coordinate efforts with other students, which is key to developing social skills and communication.

As a school based program, Higashi also provides instruction in all of the regular curricular areas. There is strong emphasis placed on special subjects, such as art and music, to build upon students' strengths and encourage their creativity. All students are given responsibility for chores at an early age, and are enrolled in various vocational training programs as they mature. A major belief is that all education should take place within as normal an environment as possible. Students participate in mainstream classes and functional activities within typical community settings.

Training in Higashi (daily life therapy)

There are no formal training programs available for professionals who are interested in this method. Information can be obtained by reading the works of the late Dr Kitahara, or by visiting one of three schools that were established according to her philosophy.

Recommended resources for Higashi (daily life therapy)

Literature

Kitahara, K. (1984) *Daily Life Therapy: A Method of Educating Autistic Children, Record of Actual Education at Musashino Higashi Gakuen School, Japan. Volumes 1–3*. Boston, MA: Nimrod Press.

Larkin, A.S. and Gurry, S. (1998) 'Brief report: Progress reported in three children with autism using Daily Life Therapy.' *Journal of Autism and Developmental Disorders, 28*, 4, 339–342.

Peacock, G. (1994) *Higashi: Implementing Daily Life Therapy in Japan. A Visit to the Musashino Higashi Gakuen School in Tokyo*. London: The National Autistic Society.

Quill, K. (1989) 'Daily Life Therapy: A Japanese model of educating children with autism.' *Journal of Autism and Developmental Disorders, 19*, 4, 625–635.

Agencies, organizations, and websites

Boston Higashi School, Inc.
800 North Main Street
Randolph, MA 02368, USA
Telephone: +1 (781) 961-0800
Website: www.bostonhigashi.org
This school, founded in 1987 by Dr Kiyo Kitahara, offers day and residential programs for individuals with autism spectrum disorders ages 3–22.

Horizon School for Autism
Blithbury Road
Rugeley, Staffordshire WS15 3JQ, UK
Telephone: +44 (0)1889 504400

Musashino Higashi Gakuen
3-25-3 Nishikubo
Musashino, Tokyo 180-0013, Japan
Telephone: +81 (1)0 422-52-2211
Website: www.musashino-higashi.org
This is the school founded by Dr Kitahara in 1964.

HIPPOTHERAPY

Hippotherapy refers to the use of horses as a therapeutic tool to address functional limitations in a wide variety of disabilities. It is a widely accepted intervention for children with cerebral palsy and other neurological dysfunctions affecting posture and motor control, but may also be effective in promoting communication skills among children with autism and learning disabilities. Hippotherapy is used as an adjunct to the traditional techniques that are provided by trained physical therapists, occupational therapists, and speech therapists. It is not considered to be a stand-alone treatment, but may be helpful as one part of an integrated treatment plan that typically incorporates principles from *sensory integration therapy* and *neurodevelopmental therapy.*

Hippotherapy is not the same thing as therapeutic riding. *Therapeutic riding* teaches riders with disabilities to be able to control a horse or horse and carriage so that they can engage in a healthy physical activity or compete in riding challenges. Although therapeutic riding may indeed produce positive functional changes in children with disabilities, it is not considered to be a formal therapeutic intervention. Hippotherapy does not actually teach the child to ride a horse. Instead, the therapist positions the child on the horse in a manner that produces a desired change in posture, muscle tone, balance, breathing, or fine motor control. Then, the horse is guided to move while the therapist analyzes the child's response to the movement. The warmth of the horse's body, combined with rhythmic movements as the horse walks, are conducive to producing changes in the child's motor control. For children who enjoy horses, and who can develop a bond with a horse, the experience also motivates them to advance their independence in communication skills with the horse and therapist, and in fine motor and self-care skills that are part of the natural experience of riding a horse.

Limited scientific research has been conducted to validate the effects of hippotherapy, but it is widely accepted among the medical and educational communities as a possible adjunctive therapy for selected children. Because it is provided by professional therapists who use it as a part of a more integrated program of therapy, it is commonly incorporated into school physical education programs, and may be covered by some third party insurance plans.

Training in hippotherapy

The therapeutic use of horses as an adjunct to traditional speech, physical, or occupational therapy is not formally regulated in either the United States or the United Kingdom. Training is available in the form of short courses, or as university level programs lasting from one to three years post qualifying in the professional discipline. Voluntary registration is available through several agencies, and signifies the completion of an approved course of training.

Recommended resources for hippotherapy

Literature

Debuse, D., Chandler, C. and Gibb, C. (2005) 'An exploration of German and British physiotherapists' views on the effects of hippotherapy and their measurement.' *Physiotherapy Theory and Practice, 21*, 4, 219–242.

Macauley, B.L. and Gutierrez, K.M. (2004) 'The effectiveness of hippotherapy for children with language learning disabilities.' *Communication Disorders Quarterly, 25*, 4, 205–213.

Meregillano, G. (2004) 'Hippotherapy.' *Physical Medicine and Rehabilitation Clinics of North America, 15*, 4, 843–854.

Potter, J.T., Evans, J.W. and Nolt, B.H. (1994) 'Therapeutic horseback riding.' *Journal of the American Veterinary Medical Association, 204*, 1, 131–133.

Scott, N. (2005) *Special Needs, Special Horses: A Guide to the Benefits of Therapeutic Riding.* Denton, TX: University of North Texas Press.

Agencies, organizations, and websites

American Hippotherapy Association, Inc.
136 Bush Road
Damascus, PA 18415, USA
Telephone: +1 (888) 851-4592
Website: www.americanhippotherapyassociation.org
This is a professional organization for therapists and others who are interested in the use of equine movement as a treatment modality.

American Hippotherapy Certification Board
Professional Testing Corporation
1350 Broadway, 17th Floor
New York, NY 10018, USA
Telephone: +1 (212) 356-0660
Website: www.ptcny.com
This is the certifying body of the American Hippotherapy Association.

The Chartered Society of Physiotherapy
14 Bedford Row
London WC1R 4ED, UK
Telephone: +44 (0)207 306 6666
Website: www.csp.org.uk
This is the professional society for physiotherapists in the United Kingdom.

Federation of Riding for the Disabled International (FRDI)
PO Box 886
WERRIBEE, Victoria 3030, Australia
Telephone: +61 (0)3 9731 7282
Website: www.frdi.net
This organization was developed to form worldwide links between countries
and centers offering therapeutic riding and driving. It promotes the
development of national and international standards of instruction and safety
when using horses for therapeutic purposes. It is involved in research and
publication around the theme of therapeutic horseback riding.

North American Riding for the Handicapped Association
PO Box 33150
Denver, CO 80233, USA
Telephone: +1 (800) 369-7433
Website: www.narha.org
This site offers extensive information about equine-assisted activities for
individuals with and without disabilities. It provides a link to its affiliate
member, the American Hippotherapy Association, and offers three levels of
instructor certification for individuals interested in teaching riding and driving.

Riding for the Disabled Association
Lavinia Norfolk House, Avenue R
Stonleigh Park, Warwickshire CV8 2LY, UK
Telephone: +44 (0)845 658 1082
Website: www.rda.org.uk
This organization is devoted to ensuring a high level of professionalism to
people with disabilities who are interested in riding and carriage driving. It
works closely with children and young adults with a wide range of special needs
through schools and colleges, and offers links to groups that offer programs
throughout the United Kingdom.

INTERACTIVE METRONOME®

The *Interactive Metronome® (IM) Program* is a brain-based treatment program that
is designed to train the brain to plan, sequence, and process information more
effectively through repetition of interactive exercises that are appropriate for
children at a developmental level of six years or older. Wearing headphones and

motion sensors, the child listens to different rhythmic beats while performing a variety of hand and foot exercises that attempt to match the beat. Computerized technology measures the accuracy of the child's responses, and provides immediate auditory feedback to guide the child to correct his or her performance. Often, IM therapy is used by occupational therapists in combination with sensory integration therapy to help children with autism spectrum disorders, ADHD, and specific learning disabilities including dyslexia. Typically, the program consists of 12 to 15 hours of treatment that can be completed in three to five weeks. Advocates suggest that the training can improve attention and concentration, motor control and coordination, language processing, reading and math fluency, and the ability to regulate aggression or impulsivity.

Training in Interactive Metronome®

Professionals from a variety of disciplines can become certified in Interactive Metronome® by purchasing and installing software for a PC and participating in an assisted self-training process that takes ten hours to complete. Two levels of certification are provided: *IMC Group Only* designation, for providers trained to work with groups of higher functioning students in schools or other institutional settings, and *IMC* designation, for providers trained to offer training in both individual and group modes.

Recommended Resources for Interactive Metronome®

Literature

Bartscherer, M.L. and Dole, R.L. (2005) 'Interactive Metronome® training for a 9-year-old boy with attention and motor difficulties.' *Physiotherapy Theory and Practice, 21*, 4, 257–269.

Koomar, J., Burpee, J.D., DeJean, V., Frick, S. Kawar, M. and Fischer, D.M. (2001) 'Theoretical and clinical perspectives on the Interactive Metronome®: A view from occupational therapy practice.' *American Journal of Occupational Therapy, 55*, 2, 163–166.

Kuhlman, K. and Schweinhart, L.J. (1999) *Timing in Child Development.* Ypsilanti, MI: High/Scope Educational Research Foundation.

Schaffer, R.J., Jacokes, L.E., Cassidy, J.F., Greenspan, S.I., Tuchman, R.F. and Stemmer Jr., P.J. (2001) 'Effect of Interactive Metronome® training on children with ADHD.' *The American Journal of Occupational Therapy, 55*, 2, 155–162.

Agencies, organizations, and websites
Interactive Metronome®
2500 Weston Road, Suite 403
Weston, FL 33331, USA
Telephone: +1 (877) 994-6776
Website: www.interactivemetronome.com
The home website of the Interactive Metronome® Program, offering
information about application, training, and research, as well as a listing of
certified providers.

MASSAGE THERAPY

Massage refers to various practices involving rubbing, pressing, tapping, or otherwise manipulating the muscles and soft tissues of the body. It is a practice that
has been used for thousands of years to promote a sense of well-being, to
relieve pain, and to produce other health effects. In fact, massage is something
that most of us do naturally, as in rubbing the forehead when we have a
headache, or squeezing or kneading a sore muscle after over exercising.

Massage therapy refers to the specific application of massage techniques for
therapeutic purposes. It is a common treatment for children with learning disabilities, autism, ADHD, and other disabilities, and is believed to produce a wide
range of benefits, including reduced stress and anxiety, improved sleep habits,
behavior, and social interaction. It is not known exactly why massage produces
these benefits. However, scientists do know that massage can increase the flow
of oxygen and blood to the part being massaged, resulting in warmth and a
decrease of pain. Studies also show that massage can decrease the production of
the stress hormone, *cortisol*, and increase the flow of the neurotransmitters
dopamine and *serotonin*, which can influence alertness and a ready state for action.

There are many, many different types of massage techniques. *Swedish massage*
uses lotions or oils along with long, smooth strokes, usually in the direction of
the heart to promote relaxation and flexibility. *Deep tissue massage* uses little or no
lubricant, and starts superficially, then progresses into the deeper layer of tissue
by using firm pressure to work on a specific joint, muscle or group of muscles.
Infant massage uses very gentle techniques, and is used to decrease stress, provide
sensory stimulation, and strengthen the immune system in infants, including
those born pre-term. *Myofascial release* (also called *trigger point therapy*) is a specialized form of physical therapy that uses the knuckles or elbows to slowly
elongate and release restrictions present in soft tissues (*fascia*) which may result
from poor posture, injury, or physical disabilities. Often, massage therapy tech-

niques are used as part of a holistic treatment approach, and may overlap with or be combined with some of the other interventions described in this book.

Massage therapy is generally considered a safe and pleasant intervention. When provided by nurses, physical therapists, or other trained professionals to promote relaxation and reduce pain, it is considered part of conventional medicine and is widely accepted as a beneficial treatment. Massage therapy as delivered by massage therapists to produce other health or behavioral effects is considered more controversial, although the scientific evidence of efficacy is growing. Side effects are few, and may include swelling or bruising of tissues, or skin sensitivity for those who may be allergic to the lubricants used. Massage should not be performed on children with fevers or active infections, open wounds, fragile skin conditions, or certain other health related concerns. The therapist should conduct an interview about potential health risks before instituting massage.

Training in massage therapy

Massage therapy is often practiced by health care professionals who are otherwise regulated by their profession, such as chiropractors, osteopaths, nurses, physical therapists, or occupational therapists. These professionals may receive training in massage as part of their professional education, or may take post-graduate continuing education courses. Numerous massage therapy schools, college programs, and training programs exist to offer training to those who lack other professional qualifications for providing massage therapy. These programs vary widely as to their accreditation status, length of training, and the specific techniques included in the instruction. Most states in the United States require massage therapists to meet state regulations for licensure, which may include a minimum number of hours of training or passing a national certification exam. Massage therapy is presently not regulated in the United Kingdom, although therapists may choose to voluntarily register with one of several organizations that acknowledge acceptable levels of training and ethical practice.

Recommended resources for massage therapy

Literature

Braun, M.B. and Simonson, S.J. (2007) *Introduction to Massage Therapy.* Philadelphia, PA: Lippincott Williams & Wilkins.

Capellini, S. (2006) *Massage Therapy: Career Guide for Hands-on-Success.* Clifton Park, NY: Thomson Delmar Learning.

Cullen-Powell, L.A., Barlow, J.H. and Cushway, D. (2005) 'Exploring a massage intervention for parents and their children with autism: The implications for bonding and attachment.' *Journal of Child Health Care, 9*, 4, 245–255.

Escalona, A., Field, T., Singer-Strunk, R., Cullen, C. and Hartshorn, K. (2001) 'Brief report: Improvements in the behavior of children with autism following massage therapy.' *Journal of Autism and Developmental Disorders, 31*, 513–516.

Field, T., Hernandez-Reif, M., Diego, M. Schanberg, S. and Kuhn, C. (2005) 'Cortisol decreases and serotonin and dopamine increase following massage therapy.' *The International Journal of Neuroscience, 115*, 10, 1397–1413.

Field, T. (2002) 'Massage therapy.' *Medical Clinics of North America, 86*, 163–171.

Hart, S., Field, T., Hernandez-Reif, M., and Lundy, B. (1998) 'Preschoolers' cognitive performance improves following massage.' *Early Child Development and Care, 143*, 59–64.

Khilnani, S., Field, T., Hernandez-Reif, M. and Schanberg, S. (2003) 'Massage therapy improves mood and behavior of students with attention-deficit/hyperactivity disorder.' *Adolescence, 38*, 623–638.

Manheim, C. (2001) *The Myofascial Release Manual, 3rd edn.* New York: Slack, Inc.

McClure, V. (2000) *Infant Massage: A Handbook for Loving Parents, Revised Edn.* New York: Bantam Books.

Agencies, organizations, and websites

American Massage Therapy Association
500 Davis Street
Evanston, IL 60201, USA
Telephone: +1 (877) 905-2700
Website: www.amtamassage.org
This is an international member-driven organization for the massage therapy profession.

General Council for Massage Therapy
27 Old Gloucester Street
London WC1N 3XX, UK
Telephone: +44 (0)870 850 4452
Website: www.gcmt.org.uk
This council offers voluntary registration of massage therapists in the United Kingdom.

International Association of Infant Massage (IAIM)
88 Copse Hill
Harlow, Essex CM19 4PP, UK
Telephone: +44 (0)1279 304455

Website: www.iaim.org.uk
This organization offers information and training specific to the use of massage with infants.

National Certification Board for Therapeutic Massage and Bodywork
1901 S. Meyers Road, Suite 240
Oakbrook Terrace, IL 60181-5243, USA
Telephone: +1 (800) 296-0664
Website: www.ncbmb.com
This is a voluntary certifying agency for massage therapists; certification is required for licensure in some states.

The Massage Therapy Institute of Great Britain
PO Box 2726
London NW2 3NR, UK
Telephone: +44 (0)20 7724 7198
Website: www.cmhmassage.co.uk
This is an educational and professional organization for massage therapists. It offers reliable research information to its members, and offers a listing of qualified members.

Touch Research Institute
University of Miami School of Medicine
Mailman Center for Child Development
1601 NW 12th Avenue, 7th Floor, Suite 7037
Miami, FL 33101, USA
Telephone: +1 (305) 243-6781
Website: www.miami.edu/touch-research
This center is devoted to the study of touch and its application in science and medicine. It offers an extensive listing of research abstracts using massage for the treatment of various disorders.

PATTERNING (DOMAN-DELACATO METHOD)

Patterning is a controversial treatment that is known by a number of names, including *psychomotor patterning, neurophysiological retraining* and the *Doman-Delacato method*. It was introduced as a treatment for children with brain injuries, especially cerebral palsy, by physical therapist Glenn Doman and educational psychologist Carl Delacato during the early 1960s at the Institutes for the Achievement of Human Potential in Philadelphia, PA. Patterning is proposed to have positive benefits for children with a wide range of disabilities, including autism, ADHD, mental retardation, and learning disabilities.

The theory behind patterning is based on the belief that children with disabilities fail to progress through the typical developmental stages of movement, and that this leads to neurological disorganization. Treatment starts by determining the child's current developmental stage of neurological organization. Then, a team of three to five people (usually volunteers) simultaneously move the child's head and limbs through a pattern of movement (such as crawling) that is typical for that particular developmental stage. The pattern must be repeated for at least five minutes, four times a day. Other techniques that may be used along with the patterning include various methods of sensory stimulation, re-breathing expired air through a face mask to increase blood flow to the brain, and limiting the intake of fluids, sugars and salts in an effort to decrease the production of cerebrospinal fluid and to reduce brain irritability. Proponents believe that if the patterning sequence is rigorously applied on a daily basis, undamaged brain cells will be programmed to take over the function of damaged brain cells, allowing the child to progress to the next developmental stage. Unfortunately, the theory has not been subjected to controlled scientific study, and the method has been harshly criticized by the medical community. Critics also express concern that the program demands an inordinate amount of time on the part of parents and volunteers, and can prevent them from pursuing other treatment options.

Training in patterning

There are no formal training programs for professionals interested in learning the theory and practice of patterning techniques. The Institute for the Achievement of Human Potential and its affiliates train employees to provide the treatments. They offer training workshops, books, and home instruction materials for parents who are interested in the method.

Recommended resources for patterning

Literature

American Academy of Pediatrics, Committee on Children with Disabilities (1999) 'Policy statement: The treatment of neurologically impaired children using patterning.' *Pediatrics, 104*, 1149–1151.

Doman, G. (1994) *What to do About Your Brain Injured Child.* Wyndmoor, PA: The Gentle Revolution Press.

Matthews, D. (1988) 'Controversial therapies in the treatment of cerebral palsy.' *Pediatric Annals, 17*, 762–764.

Novella, S. (2001) *Psychomotor patterning.* Available at www.quackwatch.org/01QuackeryRelatedTopics/patterning.html, accessed 19 February 2007.

Agencies, organizations, and websites

Delacato International
PO Box 836
Fort Washington, PA 19034, USA
Telephone: +1 (215) 233-3352
and
Delacato Centre UK
26 Gwscwm Park
Burry Port, Carmarthenshire SA16 ODX, Wales
Telephone: +44 (0)1554 834 954
Website: www.delacato.net
This website offers an overview of the Delacato method, with listings of
publications and international centers.

Institutes for the Achievement of Human Potential (IAHP)
8801 Stenton Avenue
Wyndmoor, PA 19038, USA
Telephone: +1 (215) 233-2050
Website: www.iahp.org
This is the world headquarters for IAHP. It offers links to international sites,
sponsors parent training sessions, and publishes a wide array of books and
materials for consumers.

National Association for Child Development
549 25th Street
Ogden, UT 84401-2422, USA
Telephone: +1 (801) 621-8606
Website: www.nacd.org
This association is run by Robert Doman, nephew of Glenn Doman, and
offers patterning as a part of its program for children with ADHD and brain
injuries.

REFLEXOLOGY

Reflexology, also referred to as *zone therapy*, is a specialized form of massage that is
believed to activate the body's healing power by applying firm pressure to designated areas of the feet or hands. Reflexologists believe that the body is divided
into ten longitudinal energy zones that run throughout the length of the body.
All of the organs and body parts located along the zone are believed to be connected by a flow of energy, and this energy culminates at the endpoints of the
zones, either in the feet or the hands. By feeling the patient's hands and feet, a
reflexologist diagnoses abnormalities in other parts of the body. Then, after
referring to detailed reflexology charts, the reflexologist determines what
specific part of the feet or hands require pressure to stimulate a flow of energy,

blood or nutrition to the corresponding body part. Unfortunately, there is no compelling scientific evidence that these pathways actually exist.

Reflexology treatments usually take about 45 minutes to one hour, and begin with a gentle massage of the feet to promote relaxation. After the reflexologist determines the patient's concerns, he or she applies firm pressure to designated points on both hands and feet, while the patient describes any discomfort felt elsewhere in the body. The pressure is firm enough that some patients describe it as uncomfortable. Multiple sessions may be recommended, and there are a number of reflexology products on the market, such as foot massage devices or shoe inserts, that may be suggested for use at home.

Research is limited in the field of reflexology. Proponents claim widespread benefits, including stress reduction, weight loss, improved circulation, pain relief, and curing or improving many illnesses. Most practitioners are careful to state, however, that the primary purpose of the intervention is to promote stress reduction, and that they are not primarily focused on diagnosing or treating health problems, which is the role of a licensed health practitioner. For children with special needs, it has been used to reduce hyperactivity, reduce bedwetting, promote weight loss, and improve feeding in picky eaters. It may also help to reduce oversensitivity to touch in children with autism.

Training in reflexology

The practice of reflexology is not formally regulated in either the United States or the United Kingdom, although it may be incorporated into the practice of health care professionals who are otherwise licensed or certified in their field. Most often, reflexology is learned through attendance at seminars, or is self-taught through books or distance learning programs. Voluntary certification programs are available.

Recommended resources for reflexology

Literature

Barrett, S. (2004) *Reflexology: A Close Look*. Available at www.quackwatch.org/01QuackeryRelatedTopics/reflex.html, accessed 18 January 2007

Kunz, K. and Kunz, B. (1997) *The Parent's Guide to Reflexology: Helping Your Child Overcome Illness and Injury Through Touch*. New York: Three Rivers Press.

Agencies, organizations, and websites

American Reflexology Certification Board
PO Box 5147

Gulfport, FL 33737, USA
Telephone: +1 (303) 933-6921
Website: www.arcb.net

Association of Reflexologists
5 Fore Street
Taunton, Somerset TA1 1HX, UK
Telephone: +44 (0)8705 673320
Website: www.aor.org.uk
This is a professional organization for reflexologists that lists agencies and organizations devoted to reflexology worldwide. It also provides direct links to reflexology practitioners.

British Reflexology Association
Monks Orchard, Whitbourne
Worcester WR6 5RB, UK
Telephone: +44 (0)1886 821207
Website: www.britreflex.co.uk

Children and Parent Reflexology Centre
Kailish Centre of Oriental Medicine, 7 Newcourt Street
London NW8 7AA, UK
Telephone: +44 (0)207 483 3476
Website: www.childrenandparentreflexologycentre.com
This London-based center offers specialized reflexology and parent training for children, including those with special needs.

Reflexology Association of America
PO Box 26744
Columbus, OH 43226-0744, USA
Telephone: +1 (704) 657-1695
Website: www.reflexology-usa.org

Reflexology Research
PO Box 35820
Albuquerque, NM 87176-5820, USA
Telephone: +1 (504) 344-9392
Website: www.reflexology-research.com
This website provides an extensive listing of literature, products, and links relating to reflexology.

WILBARGER PROTOCOL (THERAPEUTIC BRUSHING)

The *Wilbarger protocol*, also sometimes called the *Wilbarger brushing protocol*, is a treatment designed to reduce tactile defensiveness or oversensitivity to other types of sensory stimuli. It was developed by two occupational therapists, Patricia Wilbarger and her daughter Julia in the early 1990s. This treatment is commonly used by occupational therapists for children with learning differences as one part of a broader sensory integration therapy program, which is discussed earlier in this section. It is not intended as a "stand alone" intervention, but rather as one that takes place within a framework of supporting the child in his or her overall behavioral reactions to sensory input, and to help the child to become more independent in daily occupations.

The technique involves using a surgical scrub brush to apply deep touch pressure stimulation to the hands, arms, back, legs, and feet every 90 to 120 minutes. The brushing is done slowly, firmly and in rhythm, and feels more like a massage than brushing. A specific sequence of joint compressions and pressure to the roof of the mouth is applied immediately following brushing. The protocol is usually followed for a period of two weeks, after which the therapist will recommend a maintenance program that may involve less frequent brushings.

David Mulhall, located in London, provides a similar therapeutic brushing program, and this may be of interest to parents and professionals located in the United Kingdom.

Training in the Wilbarger protocol

Training seminars are available to therapists who wish to learn the rationale and the specific technique for this intervention. Because the intervention must be carried out throughout the child's day, the treating therapist must train and supervise other caregivers to assure that they are correctly performing the technique. Improper use of the protocol may be uncomfortable for the child, and may cause undesirable effects.

Recommended resources for the Wilbarger protocol

Literature

Foss, A., Swinth, Y., McGruder, J. and Tomlin, G. (2003) 'Sensory modulation disorder and the Wilbarger Protocol: An evidence review.' *OT Practice, 8, 12,* 1–8.

Miller, L.J. (2005) *Sensational Kids: Hope and Help for Children with Sensory Processing Disorders.* New York: G.P. Putnam's Sons.

Wilbarger, J. and Wilbarger, P. (2002) 'The Wilbarger approach to treating sensory defensiveness.' In A.C. Bundy, S.J. Lane and E.A. Murray (eds.) *Sensory Integration Theory and Practice, 2nd edn* (pp. 335–338). Philadelphia, PA: F.A. Davis.

Wilbarger, P. and Wilbarger, J. (1991) *Sensory Defensiveness in Children Aged 2–12.* Denver, CO: Avanti Educational Programs.

Agencies, organizations, and websites

Avanti Educational Programs
14547 Titus Street, Suite 109
Van Nuys, CA 91402-4918, USA
Telephone: +1 (818) 782-7366

David Mulhall Centre
31 Webbs Road
London SW11 6RU, UK
Telephone: +44 (0)207 223 4321
Website: www.davidmulhall.co.uk

The Sensory Processing Disorder Foundation
5655 S. Yosemite, Suite 305
Greenwood Village, CO 80111, USA
Telephone: +1 (303) 794-1182
Website: www.spdnetwork.org

YOGA

Yoga is an ancient Indian practice (dating to at least 3000 BC) that centers around transforming the mind to become liberated from its earthly bonds. It is often used as part of holistic health practices designed to promote physical, psychological, and spiritual health and wellness. The traditional practice of yoga includes five components: relaxation, exercise, correct breathing, a healthy diet, and meditation. There are numerous different traditions of yoga that can be practiced. In the West, the most common type of yoga is *Hatha yoga*, a form of yoga that places special emphasis on exercise poses (known as *asanas*) and correct breathing (known as *pranayama*). Yoga as practiced in the West is often considered an integral part of fitness and well-being programs. The poses used in yoga can be helpful in building muscle tone and flexibility, improving posture and balance, and promoting relaxation.

Yoga therapy refers to the adaptation of traditional yoga techniques to address specific health or psychological problems in individuals with special needs. It is conducted by yoga teachers who have received specialized training in understanding of patients with special needs, and in the selection and use of therapeutic yoga techniques.

Both yoga and yoga therapy are commonly used with children who have autism, ADHD, or other learning disabilities, and are claimed to improve body awareness, promote self-regulation, and improve attention. However, few studies have been conducted to support these claims. When yoga therapy is recommended, it may be offered in individual or group sessions. Parent training and support is important, because yoga should be practiced as a daily lifestyle routine to be effective.

Training in yoga

There are numerous opportunities to become trained as a teacher of yoga. Programs vary in their standards and the specific type of yoga that is taught. Sometimes, the practice of yoga is incorporated into the professional practice of someone with a background in therapy or education, or is used as one aspect of a holistic health practitioner's practice. Sometimes, though, yoga is instructed by someone with training in experience only in yoga. Yoga therapy is different than yoga teaching, in that the yoga is used specifically for people with physical or psychological challenges. The International Association of Yoga Therapists in association with the Yoga Alliance is attempting to develop standards for the profession, and maintains a registry of therapists who have met high standards of education in therapeutic yoga. In the United Kingdom, teachers who have trained with the British Wheel of Yoga Teachers (or a comparable program) can join the Register of Exercise Professionals, an initiative founded by the Department of Health.

Recommended resources for yoga

Literature

Bersma, D., Visscher, M., Kooistra, A. and Evans, A.M. (2003) *Yoga Games for Children: Fun and Fitness with Postures, Movements, and Breath.* Alameda, CA: Hunter House Publishers.

Betts, D.E. and Betts, S.E. (2006) *Yoga for Children with Autism Spectrum Disorders: A Step-by-Step Guide for Parents and Caregivers.* London: Jessica Kingsley Publishers.

Cuomo, N. (2007) *Integrated Yoga: Yoga with a Sensory Integrative Approach.* London: Jessica Kingsley Publishers.

Jensen, P.S. and Kenny, D.T. (2004) The effects of yoga on the attention and behavior of boys with attention deficit hyperactivity disorder (ADHD). *Journal of Attention Disorders, 7,* 4, 205–216.

Sumar, S. (1998) *Yoga for the Special Child: A Therapeutic Approach for Infants and Children with Down Syndrome, Cerebral Palsy, and Learning Disabilities.* Buckingham, VA: Special Yoga Publications.

Agencies, organizations, and websites

British Wheel of Yoga Teachers, Central Office
25 Jermyn Street
Sleaford, Lincolnshire NG34 7RU, UK
Telephone: +44 (0)1529 306851
Website: www.bwy.org.uk
This is the governing body for yoga in the United Kingdom.

International Association of Yoga Therapists
115 S. McCormick Street, Suite 3
Prescott, AZ 86303, USA
Telephone: +1 (928) 541-0004
Website: www.iayt.org
This is a non-profit organization supporting research and education in yoga to the Western world.

Yoga Alliance
7801 Old Branch Avenue, Suite 400, PO Box 369
Clinton, MD 20735, USA
Telephone: +1 (877) 964-2255
Website: www.yogaalliance.org
This organization registers both individual yoga teachers and yoga teacher training programs that meet minimal educational standards as set by the organization. They maintain a national registry of teachers who have met these standards.

Yoga Buds
47 Algers Road
Loughton, Essex IG10 4NG, UK
Telephone: +44 (0)208 508 3653
Website: www.yogabuds.org.uk
This organization offers an advanced diploma for teaching yoga to children, and is devoted to integrating yoga into the national curriculum for schools in the United Kingdom.

Yoga for the Special Child
2100 Constitution Boulevard, Suite 103
Sarasota, FL 34231, USA
Telephone: +1 (888) 900-YOGA
Website: www.specialyoga.com

Yoga for the Special Child – UK
First Floor of the Tay Building, 2a Wrentham Avenue
London NW10 3HA, UK
Telephone: +44 (0)208 968 1900
Website: www.specialyoga.org.uk
These centers specialize in providing direct services and teacher training
specifically focused on yoga for the child with special needs.

Chapter 7

ENERGY THERAPIES

CHROMOTHERAPY

Chromotherapy, also referred to as *color therapy*, or *colorology* refers to the use of color and light to balance a person's physical, emotional, spiritual, or mental energy. It is an ancient form of healing, possibly rooted in the Indian practices of Ayurveda. The belief behind chromotherapy is that colors can cause predictable mood or emotional changes in people. Most people would agree that vivid hues of red, orange, and yellow are energizing, while blue and violet are more calming hues. Color therapists associate colors with seven spiritual centers, or *chakras*, that are responsible for storing and distributing information. Each chakra is also related to one of the four primary elements: earth, air, fire and water. Each chakra is associated with a particular organ or biological system in the body, and has a dominant color. Disease or stress occurs when these colors are imbalanced.

Color therapists typically diagnose problems using *Luscher's color test*, which involves selecting colors in order of favorite to least favorite. Based on the patient's responses, the color therapist diagnoses the problem and then prescribes various uses of light and color to heal the imbalances. The application of color can take many forms, including colored fabrics or eyeglasses, bath treatments, gemstones, prisms, blinking lights, candles, etc. *Colorpuncture* is a specialized form of color therapy, developed by German acupuncturist Peter Mandel. It involves applying color and light to acupuncture points on the body.

Chromotherapy is not usually used as a primary intervention, but often complements the interventions used by holistic or natural healers. There is no real scientific evidence to support the effectiveness of this intervention.

Training in chromotherapy

The practice of chromotherapy is not formally regulated in either the United States or the United Kingdom. Most practitioners attend various workshops and other continuing education offerings, and also learn through reading books about the techniques. Voluntary registration as a color therapist is available in Britain through the Institute for Complementary Medicine.

Recommended resources for chromotherapy

Literature

Boyatzis, C.J. and Varghese, R. (1994) 'Children's emotional associations with color.' *Journal of Genetic Psychology, 155*, 1, 77–86.

Gimbel, T. (1994) *Healing with Color and Light.* New York: Simon & Schuster Books.

Gimbel, T. (2001) *Healing Color.* London: Gaia Books.

Gimbel, T. (2005) *The Healing Energies of Color.* London: Gaia Books.

Graham, H. (1998) *Discover Color Therapy.* Berkeley, CA: Ulysses Press.

Agencies, organizations, and websites

International Association of Color

Telephone: +44 (0)208 349 3299 (UK)

Website: www.iac-colour.co.uk

This is the home website for the professional organization responsible for setting standards of training and regulation of color therapy practitioners. It offers information about books and materials, offers a list of color practitioners worldwide, and lists schools/programs that offer training in color therapy worldwide.

MAGNETIC FIELD THERAPY

Magnetic field therapy uses various types of magnets to maintain health and to treat illness, especially pain. The use of magnets for treating pain and stiffness dates back to ancient medical practices in China, but was not commonly used in current medical practices until the 1990s when it was popularized for use in treating injuries and joint pain associated with playing sports. Practitioners who use this approach believe that the body's electromagnetic field must be balanced in order to maintain health and emotional well-being. Because magnets are believed to produce a slight electrical current, they may stimulate nerve endings and help release natural pain killers produced by the body. This electrical stimulation may also cause cellular reactions that result in increased blood flow and oxygenation to the tissues that are stimulated. The magnets used in this therapy may be *static*, as in magnetic bracelets, *electrically charged* to produce a pulsating current to the part of the body being treated, or used along with acupuncture or other alternative interventions to treat energy pathways in the body. Although this therapy is most widely used in the treatment of pain, it has also been suggested as an intervention that may be helpful for sleep disturbances, and for helping to promote relaxation.

Training in magnetic field therapy

The use of magnets as an adjunct for therapy is not regulated. Magnets may be purchased without prescription from many sources. Training in the use of pulsating electromagnetic therapy usually takes place through continuing education opportunities that are available to many types of practitioners.

Recommended resources for magnetic field therapy

Literature

Fernandez, M.I., Watson, P.J. and Rowbotham, D.J. (2007) 'Effect of pulsed magnetic field therapy on pain reported by human volunteers in a laboratory model of acute pain.' *British Journal of Anaesthesia*, *99*, 2, 266–269.

Markov, M.S. (2007) 'Magnetic field therapy: A review.' *Electromagnetic Biology and Medicine*, *26*, 1, 1–23.

Shupak, N.M., McKay, J.C., Nielson, W.R., Rollman, G.B., Prato, F.S. and Thomas, A.W. (2006) 'Exposure to a specific pulsed low-frequency magnetic field: A double-blind placebo-controlled study of effects on pain ratings in rheumatoid arthritis and fibromyalgia patients.' *Pain Research and Management: The Journal of the Canadian Pain Society*, *11*, 2, 85–90.

Vallbona, C. and Richards, T. (1999) 'Evolution of magnetic therapy from alternative to traditional medicine.' *Physical Medicine and Rehabilitation Clinics of North America*, *10*, 3, 729–754.

Agencies, organizations, and websites

Body Fields USA, Inc.
1645 South River Road, Suite 5
Des Plaines, Il 60018, USA
Telephone: +1 (877) 354-7152
Website: www.magnpro-usa.com
This company rents and sells products that provide pulsating electromagnetic fields for home use.

Electronic Healing
28 Keymer Road
Hassocks, West Sussex BN6 8AN, UK
Telephone: +44 (0)870 922 0068
Website: www.electronichealing.co.uk
This company sells a variety of magnetic products.

Foundation for Magnetic Science
110 South Sugan Road
New Hope, PA 18938, USA
Telephone: +1 (215) 862-6777
Website: www.magnetfoundation.org
This is an independent organization that promotes the scientific research and use of magnetic therapy.

Twister Enterprises
39 Norbert Road
Brampton, ON L6Y 2K2, Canada
Telephone: +1 (905) 453 9044
Website: www.magnetictherapycentral.com
This is a commercial provider of static magnet therapy products.

POLARITY THERAPY

Polarity therapy is a holistic approach to health and well-being that is based upon the concept of a universal life energy that is present in all humans. This approach was developed by Randolph Stone, who was trained in a number of healing arts, including osteopathic medicine, chiropractic, naturopathy, homeopathy, and Ayurvedic medicine. Stone attempted to integrate these approaches to balancing life energy, and published several books between 1947 and 1954 describing his approach. He viewed life as a spiritual journey, and believed that helping a person maintain physical and mental health was central to that journey.

The philosophy behind polarity therapy is that imbalances in the circulation of life energy can lead to mental and emotional distress, as well as to various physical ailments. A polarity therapist is trained in different methods of diagnosing and treating these imbalances, including the use of therapeutic touch, gentle body work or exercise, diet, and non-directive dialogue relating to the client's emotional state as energy is released. Sessions generally last for 60 to 90 minutes, and may be conducted weekly or every other week. The treatment is non-invasive and is considered harmless, although some of the diet recommendations, including programs designed to "detoxify" the person, could have medical implications. There is very little published research as to the scientific basis of polarity therapy, and its popularity is due primarily to anecdotal reports.

Training in polarity therapy

Polarity therapy is not regulated in either the United States or the United Kingdom. Practitioners learn the techniques through a variety of continuing education courses, which may lead to voluntary certification. Often, practitioners are trained or licensed in other professional fields and use polarity therapy as an adjunct to more traditional or to naturopathic therapies.

Recommended resources for polarity therapy

Literature

Gordon, R. (2004) *Your Healing Hands: The Polarity Experience.* Berkeley, CA: North Atlantic Books.

Mornigstar, A. (2002) *The Ayurvedic Guide to Polarity Therapy.* Twin Lakes, WI: Lotus Press.

Sills, F. (2002) *The Polarity Process.* Berkeley, CA: North Atlantic Books.

Agencies, organizations, and websites

American Polarity Therapy Association
122 N. Elm Street, Suite 512
Greensboro, NC 27401, USA
Telephone: +1 (336) 574-1121
Website: www.polaritytherapy.org
This website offers a voluntary registration program for practitioners of polarity therapy. It also offers on-line directories of schools offering training and of practitioners in the United States.

UK Polarity Therapy Association
Monomark House, 27 Old Gloucester Street
London WC1N 3XX, UK
Telephone: +44 (0)700 705 2748
Website: www.ukpta.org.uk
This website offers links to three accredited schools that offer training in polarity therapy, as well as a list of registered practitioners.

QI GONG

Qi Gong (pronounced *Chee Gung*, and sometimes spelled *Chi Kung* or *Chi Gung*) is an energy modality that originated in ancient China and is based upon traditional Chinese medical philosophy. The earliest practices occurred before recorded history and were passed down through tradition as practitioners (referred to as *Qi Gong masters*) taught and mentored new generations of masters. Qi Gong uses a vast array of postures, exercises, meditations, and breathing exercises that are designed to enhance and control the flow of *qi* (also spelled *chi*) which, according to beliefs, is the fundamental life force or energy that is responsible for maintaining one's health and vitality (see the section on acupuncture for further discussion of qi). The belief is that if qi is flowing harmoniously through all parts of the body, the body will experience a boost in the immune system. When the flow of qi is disrupted, illness results. Besides its usefulness for health maintenance, some practitioners also contend that Qi Gong can cure or prevent certain diseases, including asthma, high blood pressure, and cancer. Qi Gong sessions may be internal or external. *Internal Qi Gong* refers to the use of an exercise and breathing routine as prescribed and supervised by a Qi Gong master, while *external Qi Gong* refers to the ability of some highly skilled masters to pass their own energy to another person for the purpose of healing that person. There are thousands of different schools and forms of Qi Gong, so the specific exercises used vary according to the background, experience, and philosophy of the master. The exercises are often recommended as part of a daily routine that is used to teach self-discipline, promote health and well-being, and reduce stress. They are usually performed outdoors at the same time each morning and evening. They are performed while wearing loose clothing and no jewelry, and when the stomach is neither empty nor full. Sessions can last for minutes or hours, depending on the specific routine.

As with many traditional Chinese medical practices, there is limited scientific evidence to support these claims. This is due, in part, to the fact that qi may be thought of as a metaphysical concept, often tied to religious beliefs, and is not measurable by any existing scientific method. Despite this, Qi Gong is viewed as having potential benefit as part of an overall health maintenance routine, and may help with stress reduction, balance, flexibility, and helping to maintain muscle tone and strength. Its focus on other aspects of living a healthy lifestyle, such as a healthy diet, regular sleep, and self-discipline, is also viewed as a positive benefit of this intervention. Children who engage in these programs may show gains in self-confidence and self-esteem.

Qi Gong is often used in combination with other traditional Chinese medical interventions, especially acupuncture. Certain martial arts, including *Tai Chi* and *Kung fu*, were derived from the principles of Qi Gong and incorporate many of the same exercises. These interventions are generally considered safe for anyone who is healthy enough to engage in regular physical exercise.

Training in Qi Gong

Many schools throughout the United States and the United Kingdom offer instruction leading to becoming a teacher of Qi Gong, Tai Chi, or related martial arts. It takes many years of training and guidance from an experienced mentor to become acknowledged as a Qi Gong master. Because there are so many forms of Qi Gong, the teachings vary from one school to another, depending on the philosophy of the school. There are no generally accepted standards for training in either the United States or the United Kingdom, and the practice is not formally regulated.

Recommended resources for Qi Gong

Literature

Chu, D.A. (2004) 'Tai Chi, Qi Gong and Reiki.' *Physical Medicine and Rehabilitation Clinics of North America, 15*, 4, 774–781

Holland, A. (2000) *Voices of Qi: An Introductory Guide to Traditional Chinese Medicine.* Berkeley, CA: North Atlantic Books.

Lui, H. and Perry, P. (1997) *Mastering Miracles: The Healing Art of Qi Gong as Taught by a Master.* New York: Warner Books.

Reid, D. (1998) *A Complete Guide to Chi Gung.* Boston, MA: Shambhala.

Silva, L.M. and Cignolini, A. (2005) 'A medical qigong methodology for early intervention in autism spectrum disorder: A case series.' *The American Journal of Chinese Medicine, 33*, 2, 315–327.

Wall, R.B. (2005) 'Tai Chi and mindfulness-based stress reduction in a Boston Public Middle School.' *Journal of Pediatric Health Care, 19*, 4, 230–237.

Witt, C., Becker, M., Bandelin, K., Soellner, R. and Willich, S.N. (2005) 'Qigong for schoolchildren: A pilot study.' *Journal of Alternative and Complementary Medicine, 11*, 1, 41–47.

Agencies, organizations, and websites

International Institute of Medical Qigong
c/o Jazz Rasool MMQ
20 Greensward
Bushey, Herts WD23 4UL, UK
Telephone: +44 (0)780 108 0208
Website: www.medicalqigong.info
This is the United Kingdom branch of this organization, offering services and training in Qi Gong in England.

International Qigong Alliance
PO Box 750
Ely, MN 55731, USA
Telephone: +1 (218) 365-6330
Website: www.qigong-alliance.org
This site has links to Qi Gong instructors worldwide.

National Qigong Association
PO Box 252
Lakeland, MN 55043, USA
Telephone: +1 (888) 815-1893
Website: www.nqa.org
This organization offers four levels of volunteer certification, and also offers a large number of articles and links to other sites.

Qigong Association of America
1220 NW Kings Boulevard
Corvallis, OR 97330, USA
Telephone: +1 (541) 752-6599
Website: www.qi.org
This organization promotes awareness of Qi Gong in America, and offers many links to articles and organizations.

REIKI

Reiki is a form of *therapeutic touch* that is used to achieve a variety of health related purposes, especially reducing the effects of stress, improving mental clarity, and enhancing a sense of calmness and well-being. The term Reiki (pronounced ray-kee) is derived from the Japanese words *rei*, which means universal spirit or supreme being, and *ki*, which means the universal life force or energy. It is believed that the philosophical basis for Reiki originated in ancient Tibet. However, it became popular in the Western world during the mid-1800s when Japanese monk and physician, Mikao Usui, developed a system for Reiki, and began training others in the techniques that he promoted. Other systems of Reiki exist and various schools and practitioners vary widely as to the specific techniques they use.

All Reiki practitioners believe that ki is a spiritual force that is present and moving in all living things, and that its presence is important to all aspects of health. When the flow of ki is disrupted, an imbalance in vital energy fields results. This imbalance disrupts the body's ability to function, and leads to many different types of health problems. In performing Reiki, the practitioner channels and increases his or her own level of ki, allowing the practitioner to then serve as a conduit where ki is transferred to others. This is believed to help the patient find balance in his or her energy fields, thus promoting spiritual or physical healing. The method involves having the patient sit or lie still while fully clothed. While the patient relaxes in this position, the practitioner places his or her hands on or close to the body in various positions, and holds each position until it is determined that the flow of energy has slowed or stopped, usually after a few minutes. Some patients report that they can feel a sensation of warmth as the energy is transferred, even when the practitioner is not directly touching the patient. The number of sessions recommended varies from patient to patient, and many patients return periodically to re-balance their energy fields.

There is little scientific evidence to suggest that Reiki is an effective health intervention. However, many patients do report a feeling of deep relaxation and well-being following treatment, and there may be positive benefits to this feeling of relaxation. Critics suggest that the anecdotal reports of effectiveness reflect placebo effect on the part of highly suggestible patients.

Training in Reiki

There are no special qualifications required for people who are interested in Reiki training, although many people with other health care backgrounds seek the training. Students learn the techniques by working under the supervision of an experienced Reiki teacher or master. Depending on the particular school or system of Reiki being taught, there are three or four levels of expertise that can be achieved, and training for each level usually takes one or two days. Each level begins with an initiation phase called an *attunement* which is believed to allow the practitioner to access and open a central core of Reiki energy within the body. The process of becoming a Reiki master can take years, and requires apprenticeship with a Reiki master. In most areas of the United States and in the United Kingdom, there is no formal regulation of practicing Reiki. Some Reiki organizations are interested in pursuing voluntary standards for regulating their practice.

Recommended resources for Reiki

Literature

Chu, D.A. (2004) 'Tai Chi, Qi Gong and Reiki.' *Physical Medicine and Rehabilitation Clinics of North America, 15*, 4, 774–781.

Cullen, L. and Barlow, J. (2002) '"Kiss, cuddle, squeeze": The experiences and meaning of touch among parents of children with autism attending a Touch Therapy Programme.' *Journal of Child Health Care, 6*, 3, 171–181.

Cullen, L.A., Barlow, J.H. and Cushway, D. (2005) Positive touch, the implications for parents and their children with autism: An exploratory study. *Complementary Therapies in Clinical Practice, 11*, 3, 182–189.

Wardell, D.W. and Engebretson, J. (2001) 'Biological correlates of Reiki Touch healing.' *Journal of Advanced Nursing, 33*, 4, 439–445.

Tarborough, P.A. and Yarborough, R.T. (2005) *Children's Reiki Handbook: A Guide to Energy Healing for Kids.* Colorado Springs, CO: Andborough Publishing.

Agencies, organizations, and websites

International Association of Reiki Professionals
PO Box 6182
Nashua, NH 03063-6182, USA
Telephone: +1 (603) 881-8838
Website: www.iarp.org
This website offers resources about Reiki, including information on finding local practitioners of Reiki.

Reiki Evolution™
5 Rose Lane
Pinchbeck, Spalding, Linconshire PE11 3RN, UK
Telephone: +44 (0)845 458 3004
Website: www.reiki-evolution.co.uk
This organization offers information, on-site training courses throughout the United Kingdom, home study courses, and downloadable manuals for self-study.

The International Center for Reiki Training
21421 Hilltop Street, Unit #28
Southfield, MI 48034, USA
Telephone: +1 (208) 948-8112
Website: www.reiki.org
This website has extensive information and resources about Reiki.

The Reiki School
Telephone: +44 (0)161 980 6453
Website: www.thereikischool.co.uk
This website provides information and products pertaining to Reiki, as well as courses in Reiki throughout the United Kingdom.

THERAPEUTIC TOUCH

Therapeutic touch involves use of the hands to direct human energies in an effort to promote health, healing, and emotional well-being. It was developed during the 1970s by a nurse, Dolores Krieger, and her mentor, Dora Kunz, and has become a popular component of holistic practices in nursing, massage therapy, and other allied health therapies. This approach is based upon the belief that the human body possesses a *human energy field* that extends beyond the surface of the body. If this energy field is diminished or blocked, illness may result. Practitioners of therapeutic touch believe that they can detect this energy field by placing their hands over, but not in contact with, the patient's body, and that they can intentionally manipulate the flow of energy, thus producing healthful effects for a wide range of conditions. The therapeutic touch technique involves four steps. First, the practitioner engages in *centering*, which is a meditative process used to align the practitioner with the patient's energy level. Next, the practitioner performs an *assessment*, which involves gently sweeping the hands over or just above the patient's clothed body to detect the energy fields emanating from the patient. Proponents believe that they can detect energy through cues such as warmth or cold, or through static electricity. However, studies have consistently failed to prove the existence of a detectible human energy field. The next step involves *unruffling*, which uses circular sweeping motions to break up the patient's energy and either sweep it towards the feet and away from the body, or to redistribute to an area of lower energy. Finally, the practitioner performs an *energy transfer,* where energy is believed to pass from the practitioner to the patient. Although therapeutic touch is a widely used approach with many anecdotal reports of success, there is no credible scientific evidence to support its use as a legitimate therapeutic intervention.

Training in therapeutic touch

The use of therapeutic touch is not regulated. Several organizations offer training programs that may lead to voluntary certification. Many nursing schools incorporate training in the use of therapeutic touch into their curricula.

Recommended resources for therapeutic touch

Literature

Cullen, L.A., Barlow, J.H. and Cushway, D. (2005) 'Positive touch, the implications for parents and their children with autism: An exploratory study.' *Complementary Therapies in Clinical Practice, 11*, 3, 182–189.

Dobson, S., Upadhyaya, S., Conyers, I. and Raghavan, R. (2002) 'Touch in the care of people with profound and complex needs: A review of the literature.' *Journal of Learning Disabilities, 6,* 4, 351–362.

Hover-Kramer, D. (2001) *Healing Touch: A Guide Book for Practitioners, 2nd edn.* Clifton Park, NY: Thomson Delmar Learning.

Krieger, D. (1993) *Accepting Your Power to Heal: The Personal Practice of Therapeutic Touch.* Santa Fe, NM: Bear and Company.

Kunz, D. and Krieger, D. (2004) *The Spiritual Dimension of Therapeutic Touch.* Sanat Fe, NM: Bear and Company.

Winstead-Fry, P. and Kijek, J. (1999) 'An integrative review and meta-analysis of therapeutic touch research.' *Alternative Therapies in Health and Medicine, 5,* 6, 58–67.

Agencies, organizations, and websites

British Association of Therapeutic Touch
Broadview, 13 Constitution Hill
Ipswich IP1 3RG, UK
Website: www.ttouch.org.uk

Nurse Healers–Professional Associates International
Box 419
Craryville, NY 12521, USA
Telephone: +1 (518) 325-1185
Website: www.therapeutic-touch.org
This is the official organization of the Krieger and Kunz Therapeutic Touch (KKTT) approach, offering products, links to qualified practitioners, and training leading to certification in the approach.

ZERO BALANCING

Zero balancing is a hands-on method that attempts to balance body energy with body structure through the use of touch. It was designed by the American osteopathic physician Fritz Smith in 1973, and represents the integration of Eastern medicine's views on energy with Western views of science and body mechanics. The theory behind this approach is that the skeletal system of the body holds the most energy because of the density of the bones. Zero balancing therapists use a variety of manipulative techniques to release the energy that is stored in the bones. This is believed to balance and create stronger energy fields in the mind and body. Proponents claim that the results of this intervention include improved ability to cope with stress, an increased sense of well-being, and a reduction of the physical and mental symptoms of stress. A variety of practitioners may use this approach, but it is especially popular among chiropractors, osteopaths, and massage therapists.

Therapy begins with evaluating the musculoskeletal system for range of motion in the joints. The presence of too much or too little range of motion suggests imbalance. While the patient is fully clothed, the therapist positions the body in such a way as to promote appropriate joint motion and to allow energy to flow more smoothly. This is known as using *fulcrums*. Next, the therapist applies pressure to areas called *pivotal points*, which are energy pathways in the body. The therapist continually assesses the flow of energy through touch techniques, and adjusts the position and pressure accordingly. Other techniques are used that allow the therapist to transmit energy from him or herself, or from others, into the body of the client. As with other energy therapies, there has been little scientific study to show the effectiveness of this approach.

Training in zero balancing

A number of courses and workshops are available through the Zero Balancing Health Association and its affiliates. Voluntary certification is available and requires 100 hours of lecture and 50 hours of practicum experience.

Recommended resources for zero balancing

Literature

Barnet, J.W. (2002) 'Zero balancing: Step outside the frame.' *Massage Therapy Journal*, 41, 2, 62.

Hamwee, J. (2000) *Zero Balancing: Touching the Energy of Bone*. Berkeley, CA: North Atlantic Books.

Ralston, A.L. (1998) 'Zero Balancing: Information on a therapy.' *Complementary Therapies in Nursing and Midwifery*, 4, 2, 47–49.

Smith, F.F. (2005) *The Alchemy of Touch: Moving Towards Mastery Through the Lens of Zero Balancing*. Taos, NM: Complementary Medicine Press.

Agencies, organizations, and websites

Zero Balancing Association UK
10 Victoria Grove
Bridport, Dorset DT6 3AA, UK
Telephone: +44 (0)1308 420 007
Website: www.zerobalancinguk.org
This website offers a listing of therapists certified in zero balancing techniques who offer services in the United Kingdom.

Zero Balancing Health Association
Kings Contrivance Village Center
8640 Guilford Road, Suite 240
Columbus, MD 21046, USA
Telephone: +1 (410) 381-8956
Website: www.zerobalancing.com
This website offers general information about zero balancing as well as training/certification programs, a listing of practitioners in the United States, and books and other products.

PART 3

RESOURCES FOR CHILDREN WITH AUTISM, ATTENTION DEFICIT DISORDERS, AND OTHER LEARNING DISABILITIES

Chapter 8

RECOMMENDED READING ABOUT COMPLEMENTARY AND ALTERNATIVE MEDICINE

BOOKS

Alecson, D.G. (1999) *Alternative Treatments for Children within the Autism Spectrum: Effective, Natural Solutions for Learning Disorders, Attention Deficits, and Autistic Behaviors.* Los Angeles, CA: Keats Publishing.

Arnold, L.E. (2002) 'Treatment alternatives for attention-deficit/hyperactivity disorders.' In P.J. Jensen and J. Cooper (eds) *Attention-deficit/Hyperactivity Disorders: State of the Science and Best Practice.* Kingston, NJ: Civic Research.

Charman, R.A. (2000) *Complementary Therapies for Physical Therapists.* Oxford; Boston: Butterworth-Heinemann

Chivers, M. (2006) *Dyslexia and Alternative Therapies.* London: Jessica Kingsley Publishers.

Cummings, A., Simpson, K. and Brown, D. (2006) *Complementary and Alternative Medicine: An Illustrated Colour Text.* London: Churchill Livingstone.

Davis, C.M. (1994) *Complementary Therapies in Rehabilitation.* Thorofare, NJ: Slack, Inc.

Dillard, J. and Ziporin, T. (1998) *Alternative Medicine for Dummies.* Foster City, CA: IDG Books.

Ernst, E. (2007) *Healing, Hype, or Harm? The Debate About Complementary and Alternative Medicine.* London: Hammersmith Press.

Graham, H. (1998) *Complementary Therapies in Context: The Psychology of Healing.* London: Jessica Kingsley Publishers.

Jacobson, J.W., Foxx, R.M. and Mulick, J.A. (eds.) (2005) *Controversial Therapies for Developmental Disabilities: Fad, Fashion and Science in Professional Practice.* Mahwah, NJ: Lawrence Erlbaum Associates.

Lake, J.H. and Spiegel, D. (2006) *Complementary and Alternative Treatments in Mental Health Care.* Washington, DC: American Psychiatric Publications, Inc.

Lawton, S.C. (2007) *Asperger Syndrome: Natural Steps Toward a Better Life for You or Your Child (Complementary and Alternative Medicine).* Westport, CT: Praeger Publishers.

Mantle, F. (2007) *Complementary and Alternative Medicine for Health Professionals: A Practical Handbook.* London: Churchill Livingstone.

Pauc, R. (2007) *Brain Food Plan: Helping Your Child Overcome Learning Disabilities Through Exercise and Nutrition.* London: Virgin Books.

Stozier, A.L. and Carpenter, J. (2007) *An Introduction to Complementary and Alternative Medicine.* New York: Haworth Press.

World Health Organization (2001) *Legal Status of Traditional Medicine and Complementary/Alternative Medicine: A Worldwide Review.* Geneva: WHO (can be reviewed online at: www.complementarymedicines.com)

JOURNAL ARTICLES

Astin, J.A. (1998) 'Why patients use alternative medicine: Results of a national study.' *Journal of the American Medical Association, 279,* 19, 1548–1553.

Baumgaertel, A. (1999) 'Alternative and controversial treatments for attention-deficit/hyperactivity disorder.' *Pediatric Clinics of North America, 46,* 5, 977–992.

Berman, B.M., Singh, B.K., Lao, L., Singh, B.B., Ferentz, K.S. and Hartnoll, S.M. (1995) 'Physicians' attitudes towards complementary or alternative medicine: A regional survey.' *Journal of the American Board of Family Practitioners, 8,* 361–366.

Breuner, C.C. (2002) 'Complementary medicine in pediatrics: A review of acupuncture, homeopathy, massage, and chiropractic therapies.' *Current Problems in Pediatric and Adolescent Health Care, 32,* 10, 353–384.

Brown, K.A. and Patel, D.R. (2005) 'Complementary and alternative medicine in developmental disabilities.' *Indian Journal of Pediatrics, 72,* 11, 949–952.

Brue, A.W. and Oakland, T.D. (2002) 'Alternative treatments for attention deficit/hyperactivity disorders: Does evidence support their use?' *International Journal of Integrative Medicine, 4,* 4, 28–30, 32–35.

Cleary-Guida, M.B., Okvat, H.A., Oz, M. and Ting, W. (2001) 'A regional survey of health insurance coverage for complementary and alternative medicine: Current status and future ramifications.' *Journal of Alternative and Complementary Medicine, 7,* 3, 269–273.

Cohen, M.H. and Kemper, K.J. (2005) 'Complementary therapies in pediatrics: A legal perspective.' *Pediatrics, 115,* 3, 774–780.

Committee on Children with Disabilities (2001) 'Counseling families who choose complementary and alternative medicine for their child with chronic illness or disability.' *Pediatrics, 107,* 3, 598–599.

Eisenberg, D.M., Kessler, R., Foster, C., Norlock, F., Calkins, D. and Delbanco, T. (1993) 'Unconventional medicine in the United States: Prevalence, costs, and patterns of use.' *New England Journal of Medicine, 328*, 246–252.

Geigle, P. and Galantino, M.L. (2006) 'Survey of complementary and alternative medicine inclusion within physical therapy curricula.' *Physical Therapy*, American Physical Therapy Association. Available at www.apta.org/am/abstracts/pt2005/, accessed 25 October 2007.

Hanson, E., Kalish, L.A., Bunce, E., *et al.* (2007) 'Use of complementary and alternative medicine among children diagnosed with autism spectrum disorder.' *Journal of Autism and Developmental Disorders, 37*, 4, 628–636.

Hyman, S.L. and Levy, S.E. (2005) 'Introduction: Novel therapies in developmental disabilities – hope, reason, and evidence.' *Mental Retardation Research Reviews, 11*, 2, 107–109.

Jean, D. and Cyr, C. (2007) 'Use of complementary and alternative medicine in a general pediatric clinic.' *Pediatrics, 120*, 1, e138–141.

Kemper, K.J. (2001) 'Complementary and alternative medicine for children: Does it work?' *Archives of Diseases in Childhood, 84*, 1, 6–9.

Levy, S.E. and Hyman, S.L. (2005) 'Novel treatments for autistic spectrum disorders.' *Mental Retardation Research Reviews, 11*, 2, 131–142.

Madsen, H., Andersen, S., Nielsen, R.G., Dolmer, B.S., Høst, A. and Damkier, A. (2003) 'Use of complementary/alternative medicine among paediatric patients.' *European Journal of Pediatrics, 162*, 5, 334–342.

Maha, N. and Shaw, A. (2007) 'Academic doctors' views of complementary and alternative medicine (CAM) and its role within the NHS: An exploratory qualitative study.' *BMC Complementary and Alternative Medicine, 7*, 17.

Nickel, R.E. and Gerlach, E.K. (2001) 'The use of complementary and alternative therapies by families of children with chronic conditions and disabilities.' *Infants and Young Children, 14*, 1, 67–78.

Nickel, R.E. (1996) 'Controversial therapies for young children with developmental disabilities.' *Infants and Young Children, 8*, 4, 29–40.

Pelletier, K.R. and Astin, J.A. (2002) 'Integration and reimbursement of complementary and alternative medicine by managed care and insurance providers: 2000 update and cohort analysis.' *Alternative Therapies in Health and Medicine, 8*, 1, 38–39, 42, 44.

Pilkington, K. (2007) 'Searching for CAM evidence: An evaluation of therapy-specific search strategies.' *Journal of Alternative and Complementary Medicine, 13*, 4, 451–459.

Rojas, N.L. and Chan, E. (2005) 'Old and new controversies in the alternative treatment of attention-deficit hyperactivity disorder.' *Mental Retardation and Developmental Disability Research Reviews, 11*, 2, 116–130.

Sawni, A. and Thomas, R. (2007) 'Pediatricians' attitudes, experience, and referral patterns regarding complementary and alternative medicine: A national survey.' *BMC Complementary and Alternative Medicine, 7*, 18.

Sibinga, E.M., Ottolini, M.C., Duggan, A.K. and Wilson, M.H. (2004) 'Parent-pediatrician communication about complementary and alternative medicine use for children.' *Clinical Pediatrics, 43*, 4, 367–373.

Spigelblatt, L.S. (1995) 'Alternative medicine: Should it be used by children?' *Current Problems in Pediatrics, 25*, 180–188.

Stubberfield, T.G., Wray, T.A. and Parry, T.S. (1999) 'Utilization of alternative therapies in attention deficit hyperactivity disorder.' *Journal of Pediatrics and Child Health, 35*, 450–453.

Walcraft, J. (1999) 'Complementary therapies.' *Mental Health and Learning Disabilities Care, 2*, 10, 351–354.

Wong, H.H. and Smith, R.G. (2006) 'Patterns of complementary and alternative medical therapy use in children diagnosed with autism spectrum disorders.' *Journal of Autism and Developmental Disorders, 36*, 7, 901–909.

Chapter 9

AGENCIES, ORGANIZATIONS, AND WEBSITES

COMPLEMENTARY AND ALTERNATIVE MEDICINE

American Holistic Medical Association (AHMA)
PO Box 2016
Edmonds, WA 98020, USA
Telephone: +1 (425) 967-0737
Website: www.holisticmedicine.org
This organization offers a variety of resources for consumers and professionals, including a directory of holistic medical practitioners in the United States.

Australian Council Against Health Fraud
PO Box 1166
Paramatta NSW 2124, Australia
Telephone: +61•(0)407 959 261
Website: www.acahf.org.au

British Complementary Medicine Association
PO Box 5122
Bournemouth BH8 0WG, UK
Telephone: +44 (0)845 345 5977
Website: www.bcma.co.uk
This organization offers extensive resources, including descriptions of various therapies, directories of licensed practitioners, and links to schools that offer training.

Cochrane Collaboration
Summertown Pavillion, 18–24 Middle Way
Oxford 0X2 7LG, UK
Telephone: +44 (0)1865 310138
Website: www.cochrane.org
This is the website which collects evidence-based health care research.

Directory of Information Resources Online
Website: http://dirline.nlm.nih.gov
This website is compiled by the National Library of Medicine in the United States, and lists locations and descriptive information about a wide variety of health care organizations, including CAM associations and organizations.

Federation of Holistic Therapists
18 Shakespeare Business Centre, Hathaway Close
Eastleigh, Hampshire SO50 4SR, UK
Telephone: +44 (0)870 420 2022
Website: www.fht.org.uk
This organization was developed to help holistic therapists to improve and regulate their practice.

Henry Spink Foundation
c/o Montgomery Swann, Scotts Sufferance Wharf
1 Mill Street, London SE1 2DE, UK
Website: www.henryspink.org
This individual charity was developed to assist families of children with severe disabilities to learn more about various diagnoses and to find links to alternative treatments.

Institute for Complementary Medicine
Unit 25, Tavern Quay Business Centre
Sweden Gate, London SE16 7QZ, UK
Telephone: +44 (0)207 231 5855
Website: www.i-c-m.org.uk
This organization is a registered charity that provides public information on all aspects of safe and best practices of complementary medicine. It publishes a quarterly journal that is available online, and administers the British Register of Complementary Practitioners (BRCP).

Myomancy Foundation
Website: www.myomancy.com
This website offers a comprehensive database of articles relating to treatments available for autism, ADD and learning disabilities.

National Center for Complementary and Alternative Medicine
PO Box 7923
Gaithersburg, MD 20898-7923, USA
Telephone: +1 (888) 644-6226 (United States)
         +1 (301) 519-3153 (International)
Website: http://nccam.nih.gov

National Council Against Health Fraud, Inc.
PO Box 1276
Loma Linda, CA 92354-1276, USA
Telephone: +1 (909) 824-4838
Website: www.ncahf.org
This is a private, non-profit, voluntary health care agency that focuses upon health misinformation and fraud as public health concerns. It publishes position papers on various forms of complementary and alternative medical practices.

Natural Healers
Website: www.naturalhealers.com
This website offers an extensive listing of schools in North America that offer training in complementary and alternative medical approaches.

Pediatric Integrative Medicine Education Project
Website: www.holistickids.org
This website is designed to provide information and resources for health care providers on complementary and alternative medicine.

The Alternative Medicine Homepage
Charles B. Wessel, MLS
Falk Library of the Health Sciences
University of Pittsburgh
Pittsburgh, PA 15261, USA
Website: www.hsls.pit.edu
This website offers extensive linkages to worldwide agencies and organizations focusing on alternative medical practices.

CHILDREN, INCLUDING CHILDREN WITH DEVELOPMENTAL DISABILITIES

Ability.org
16 Almond Close
Penwortham, Preston PR1 0YQ, UK
Website: www.ability.org.uk
This website provides an extensive listing of links to disability related topics.

American Academy of Pediatrics (AAP)
141 Northwest Point Boulevard
Elk Grove Village, IL 60007, USA
Telephone: +1 (847) 434-4000
Website: www.aap.org
In addition to offering general information about children from birth through age 21, this organization offers research reports, policy and technical reports relating to complementary and alternative medicine.

American Association of Mental Retardation (AAMR)

444 North Capitol Street NW, Suite 846
Washington, DC 20001-1512, USA
Telephone: +1 (202) 387-1968 or +1 (800) 424-3688
Website: www.aamr.org
This organization promotes progressive policies, sound research, effective practices, and universal human rights for people with intellectual and developmental disabilities.

American Occupational Therapy Association (AOTA)

4720 Montgomery Lane, PO Box 31220
Bethesda, MD 20824-1220, USA
Telephone: +1 (301) 652-2682
Website: www.aota.org
This is the professional membership organization of occupational therapists. It provides public education and referrals for occupational therapy services.

American Physical Therapy Association (APTA)

1111 North Fairfax Street
Alexandria, VA 22314-1488, USA
Telephone: +1 (703) 684-2782 or +1 (800) 999-2782
Website: www.apta.org
This is the official membership website for physical therapists in the United States, and offers a variety of consumer resources.

American Psychological Association (APA)

750 First Street NE
Washington, DC 20002-4242, USA
Telephone: +1 (202) 336-5500 or +1 (800) 374-2721
Website: www.apa.org
This scientific and professional organization represents psychology in the United States. It offers a searchable database of documents relating to the field of psychology that is available through libraries, or online for a fee.

American Speech-Language Hearing Association (ASHA)

10801 Rockville Pike
Rockville, MD 20852, USA
Telephone: +1 (800) 638-8255
Website: www.asha.org
This is the professional, scientific and credentialing association for members and affiliates who are speech-language therapists, audiologists, and speech, language and hearing scientists in the United States.

Association of University Centers on Disabilities (AUCD)

1010 Wayne Avenue, Suite 920
Silver Spring, MD 20910, USA

Telephone: +1 (301) 588-8252
Website: www.aucd.org
This is the home organization for University Centers for Excellence in Developmental
Disabilities, which are supported by federal legislation in the United States, and serve as
the bridge between the academic arena and public policy and service. These centers
focus on research, training of advanced level practitioners, dissemination of
state-of-the-art knowledge, and in some cases, direct service for patients with
developmental disabilities.

Autism Independent UK
Website: www.autismuk.com
This useful website offers many information resources for parents and professionals,
including an extensive listing of links to worldwide websites relating to autism.

Autism Society of America
7910 Woodmont Avenue, Suite 300
Bethesda, MD 20814-3067, USA
Website: www.autism-society.org
This agency provides a range of information and referral services for children with
autism.

CHADD National
8181 Professional Place, Suite 150
Landover, MD 20785, USA
Telephone: +1 (800) 233-4050
Website: www.chadd.org
This organization sponsors support groups for parents of children with ADHD, and
provides continuing education programs for parents and professionals.

Children's Defense Fund
25 E. Street NW
Washington, DC 20001, USA
Telephone: +1 (202) 628-8787
Website: www.childrensdefense.org
This agency provides information about legislation pertaining to child health, welfare,
and education. It publishes a consumer guide describing parent rights under the
Individuals with Disabilities Education Act.

Council for Exceptional Children
1110 North Glebe Road, Suite 300
Arlington, VA 22201, USA
Telephone: +1 (888) 232-7733
Website: www.cec.sped.org
This is an Association for parents and professionals with an interest in children with
developmental differences. It provides literature reviews, referrals, and computer
searches.

Developmental Delay Resources
5801 Beacon Street
Pittsburgh, PA 15217, USA
Telephone: +1 (800) 497-0944
Website: www.devdelay.org
This organization serves as a clearinghouse on alternative approaches to educational and medical treatment of children with special needs.

Educational Resources Information Center (ERIC)
Website: www.eric.ed.gov
Sponsored by the Institute of Education Sciences (IES) of the United States Department of Education, this website produces the world's premier database of journal and non-journal education literature, with many full-text materials offered to consumers at no charge.

Future Horizons, Inc.
721 West Abram Street
Arlington, TX 76013, USA
Telephone: +1 (800) 489-0727
Website: www.futurehorizons-autism.com
This organization offers extensive listings of publications and continuing education opportunities relating to autism. It also offers useful links to other autism-related websites.

International Dyslexia Association
40 York Road, 4th Floor
Baltimore, MD 21204-5202, USA
Telephone: +1 (410) 296-0232
Website: www.interdys.org
This organization was formerly called the *Orton Dyslexia Society*. It promotes literacy through research, education, and advocacy.

LD Online
WETA Public Television, 2775 S. Quincy Street
Arlington, VA 22206, USA
Website: www.ldonline.org
This website offers comprehensive information about learning disabilities and ADHD geared towards all audiences, including parents, teachers, and children.

Learning Disabilities Association of America (LDA)
4156 Library Road
Pittsburgh, PA 15234-1349, USA
Telephone: +1 (412) 341-1515
Website: www.ldanatl.org

This organization disseminates information, provides advocacy, and seeks to improve education opportunities for individuals with learning disabilities.

National Autistic Society

393 City Road
London EC1V 1NG, UK
Telephone: +44 (0)207 833 2299
Website: www.nas.org.uk
This organization offers resources and services for children with autism and their families residing in the United Kingdom.

National Center for Learning Disabilities

381 Park Avenue South, Suite 1401
New York, NY 10016, USA
Telephone: +1 (212) 545-7510
Website: www.ncld.org
This agency provides public awareness of learning disabilities by publishing a magazine for parents and professionals, and by providing computer-based information and referral services.

National Dissemination Center for Children with Disabilities (NICHCY)

PO Box 1492
Washington, DC 20013, USA
Telephone: +1 (800) 695-0285 (voice and TTY)
Website: www.nichcy.org

National Education Association (NEA)

1201 16th Street NW
Washington, DC 20036-3290, USA
Telephone: +1 (202) 883-4000
Website: www.nea.org
This professional employee organization is committed to advancing the cause of public education in the United States, and offers a variety of resources to parents and professionals.

National Health Service, Customer Service Centre

The Department of Health, Richmond House
79 Whitehall, London SW1A 2NL, UK
Telephone: +44 (0)207 210 4850
Website: www.nhs.uk
The official site of the British National Health Service.

National Institute on Deafness and Other Communication Disorders

National Institutes of Health, 31 Center Drive, MSC 2320
Bethesda, MD 20892-2320, USA

Telephone: +1 (800) 241-1044
Website: www.nidcd.nih.gov
This organization maintains a directory of other organizations that can answer
questions and provide printed or electronic information on autism and communication.

National Organization for Competency Assurance (NOCA)

2020 M Street N.W., Suite 800
Washington, DC 20036, USA
Telephone: +1 (202) 367-1165
Website: www.noca/org
This organization sets quality standards for professional credentialing organizations, and
is home to the National Commission for Certifying Agencies (NCCA) which oversees
the certification of numerous health care related professions.

PubMed

Website: www.ncbi.nlm.nih.gov/literature
This is a comprehensive medical database offered free of charge through the National
Library of Medicine in the United States.

Royal College of Speech and Language Therapists

2 White Hart Yard
London SE1 1NX, UK
Telephone: +44 (0)207 378 1200
Website: www.rcslt.org
This organization represents speech and language therapists and support workers. It
aims to promote excellence in practice, and to influence health, education, and social
care policy.

Zero to Three: National Center for Infants, Toddlers, and Families

Eastern Office: 2000 M Street NW, Suite 200
Washington, DC 20036, USA
Telephone: +1 (202) 638-1144
Western Office: 350 South Bixtel, Suite 150
Los Angeles, CA 90017, USA
Telephone: +1 (213) 481-7279
Website: www.zerotothree.org
This is a national, nonprofit, multidisciplinary organization that serves to inform,
educate, and support adults who influence the lives of infants and toddlers.

SUBJECT INDEX

AUTHOR INDEX